Don't Grow Old, Grow Healthy

Don't Grow Old, Grow Healthy

Dr. Chauchard's 30-Day Rejuvenation Program

Dr. Claude Chauchard

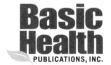
Basic Health PUBLICATIONS, INC.

The information contained in this book is based upon the research and personal and professional experiences of the author. It is not intended as a substitute for consulting with your physician or other healthcare provider. Any attempt to diagnose and treat an illness should be done under the direction of a healthcare professional.

The publisher does not advocate the use of any particular healthcare protocol but believes the information in this book should be available to the public. The publisher and author are not responsible for any adverse effects or consequences resulting from the use of the suggestions, preparations, or procedures discussed in this book. Should the reader have any questions concerning the appropriateness of any procedures or preparation mentioned, the author and the publisher strongly suggest consulting a professional healthcare advisor.

Basic Health Publications, Inc.
28812 Top of the World Drive
Laguna Beach, CA 92651
949-715-7327

Library of Congress Cataloging-in-Publication Data
Chauchard, Claude.
   [30 jours 10 ans de moins sans chirurgie. English]
   Don't grow old, grow healthy : a 30-day rejuvenation program /
Dr. Claude Chauchard.
     p. cm.
   Includes bibliographical references and index.
   ISBN-13: 978-1-59120-172-4 (alk. paper)
   ISBN-10: 1-59120-172-1
  1. Rejuvenation—Popular works. 2. Aging—Prevention—Popular works.
3. Self-care, Health—Popular works. I. Title.

   RA776.75.C47313   2006
   613—dc22

                      2006003539

Editor: John Anderson • Copyeditor: Tara Durkin
Typesetting/Book design: Gary A. Rosenberg • Cover design: Mike Stromberg

Printed in the United States of America

10   9   8   7   6   5   4   3   2   1

Contents

Acknowledgments

I started this book during the Second World Congress of Age-Preventive Medicine in Paris, which brought together several thousand doctors from around the world—proof of the vitality of this new branch of medicine. My thanks go to the organizers, especially Catherine d'Ecuyper and Christophe Luino, who had the foresight to assemble this world conference, which has already become an institution after only two years. As a result of the enthusiasm for age-preventive medicine, we can only hope that each of us will live healthier, longer lives.

Thanks also to doctors Jean-Jacques Legrand, Ronald Klatz, and Robert Goldman for their tireless encouragement in this movement.

Finally, thanks to all my family, my many collaborators, and all those friends who support me in my work and my ideas.

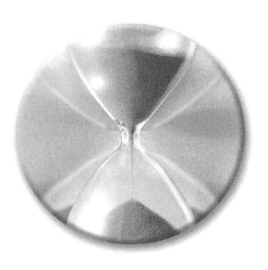

Introduction

You can find guidebooks to every country and every city in the world, to every natural phenomenon, to everything that appears foreign to us and requires detailed explanation. But before rushing off to the other side of the world to study the life cycle of the mushroom or the Minoan ruins in Crete, I suggest that you first learn to understand yourself. It is the simplest and yet most ambitious of subjects—simplest because it seems obvious, natural, a given, yet the most ambitious because the stakes are highest. We need to learn about our body so that we can live better, longer, and more youthfully.

This book is not a theoretical lesson on the human body. It is your guide to becoming younger—quickly. Learning about the body as it is taught in science classes will not do. Teachers will tell you how to distinguish between the tibia and the kneecap, the pancreas and the stomach, the right side of the brain and the left side of the brain, but will you know your body any better as a result? Will you know Rome any better if I tell you that St. Peter's Square is not in the same place as the Basilica of San Giovanni in Laterano, or that the Trevi Fountain is not by Bernini but Salvi? The problem with this approach lies in its static nature. Our science books, like those of our children, fail to take account of the fundamental issue—movement. I am referring to movement of the body, which evolves endlessly, and movement in our methods of understanding the body, which are evolving more and more quickly. This "movement of the body" is aging, while the "movement in our methods of understanding" is age-preventive medicine.

A QUESTION OF BALANCE

Vitality is basically a question of balance. There should be a balance between hormones, firstly—between catabolic hormones, which destroy the muscle and the bones, and anabolic hormones, which create and assemble proteins to form bones and muscles; that is, between the hormone cortisol (catabolic) on the one hand, and sex and growth hormones (anabolic) on the other. Up to puberty, we see the phenomenon of anabolism in development and growth. Puberty, then, is when the body begins to secrete sex and growth hormones and the level of cortisol is low. Next comes the age of maturity, with growth and sex hormones at the same level as that of cortisol. Finally, in the declining stage, the level of cortisol increases while that of the anabolic hormones decreases.

Age-preventive medicine is based partly upon the theory of hormone replacement, that is, replacing hormones that have become depleted as part of the normal aging process. However, apart from this introductory reminder, we won't discuss hormones. This subject has already been dealt with extensively. I will talk to you instead about something new, a unique and revolutionary program that could change your life with immediate effect.

As I see it, our life is made up of two slopes: the upward slope of growth until around the age of thirty, followed by the period of maturity until the age of fifty or sixty, and then a downward slope until the end, which we hope will be as late as possible, especially if you wish to prolong your vitality! It is this second slope that we need to imagine differently, especially if the first upward slope has been satisfactory in medical terms. I believe that there is a programmed and normal form of the aging process, but also an accelerated form of aging that depends on the behavior of each individual.

How should we go about entering into this second stage of our life? How can we achieve the state of perfect balance? Follow this guide: it will reveal to you new secrets of youthfulness, important information that you have never heard of, and recent scientific research in the fight against aging.

THE JOURNEY TO HEALTH

This book is a travel guide to help you discover your body the way you discover a town: the lively areas, the good addresses, the things you mustn't miss, and what to take with you. The journey should take about a month, the length of time generally considered appropriate for travellers to really get to know a town—but a record time for mastering your body and achieving youthfulness.

In the beginning of this journey, I will tell you about inflammation of cell membranes. I will explain what this inflammatory reaction is, how it is released in the body, what the causes are, and why these cell membranes made of good fatty acids oxidize, harden, and decay. Inflammation is a dominant factor in cellular aging, and is followed by six other related phenomena that provoke inflammatory damage: insulin resistance, food allergies, oxidation, glycation, fatty acids, and stress. Targeting these inflammatory phenomena with nutrition and other natural therapies represents the new approach to age prevention revealed in this guide.

My intention is to give you concrete ideas that can be immediately put into practice. To prove the efficacy of what I am recommending, I will suggest that you follow a short program of ideal nutrition for just four days, which will allow you to regenerate your cells, in particular, the cells of your face. This is what I call the "fresh face" program. This brief program combines anti-inflammatory nutrition, foods that fight free radicals, anti-glycation, insulin regulation, and micronutrition. Later, with the full program, you will eliminate the years as never before. This program repairs all the cells of the human organism—that is why it is unique and exceptional.

I will reveal to you my best prescriptions and my shocking discoveries on aging. Today, we can live until 120 and maybe beyond. My advice will teach you to prolong your vitality. This program can help you reclaim ten years in just thirty days. You risk nothing, except becoming younger. Go for it. Go along with my ideas, and take a little time until the penny drops, as they say in Belgium.

So, follow the guide . . .

HOW TO USE THIS BOOK

First, I will ask you to take a preliminary test aimed at determining your "aptitude" for staying young. It will establish the idea of age prevention and let you know where you stand in terms of managing your "health capital." By reading certain parameters, we can establish the "biological" or "real" age of the body, which should be more or less in line with our chronological age. This test serves as an orientation and leads to a personal interrogation but is no substitute for more in-depth examinations covered in the rest of the book.

The chapters that follow the test are in the form of an extended conversation with me conducted by a patient named Julien. The question-and-answer format allows you to discover and understand, one by one, the true causes of aging and how to take control of them. The discussions concentrate on the factor of inflammation, which is undoubtedly at the crossroads of these causes. At the end of this material, you will finally understand what inflammation is and how to fight against free radicals, glycation, and insulin excess. I will explain what lies behind these academic terms and how to correct their detrimental effects with practical advice and the help of new medicines that restore balance to the body.

Two healthy nutrition courses are proposed in the book—a short one of four days to familiarize you with the method and test out my theories (Chapter 3), and another more ambitious course, my 30-Day Timely Nutrition Vitality Program (Chapter 10). In just a few days, you can change your appearance and look at the improvement in the mirror. You'll see the difference almost immediately—you will appear younger with fewer wrinkles, and have soft skin, a clear complexion, and less visible crow's-feet.

I will also help you identify everyday methods for preventing, rather than accepting, aging:

- Advice on your everyday eating

- Practical tips and daily habits you should adopt

- Sensible advice to feel well physically, psychologically, and spiritually

I invite you to send me an e-mail at drchauchard@hotmail.com to let me know how my program worked for you, or to express any doubts you may have. Your feedback will help my research, and, of course, I will do my best to answer your questions.

The Stay Young Aptitude Test

Growing old is not a slope that everyone
descends at the same speed.
It is an irregular flight of stairs that some
tumble down faster than others.

—SIMONE DE BEAUVOIR, FROM *LA VIEILLESSE* (PARIS: GALLIMARD, 1970)

We don't all age the same way. This inequality between individuals has led scientists to determine biological markers to measure the age of our body, or our "health capital." The health questions that follow concern the bones, hormonal balance, sight, lungs, exercise, the blood system, and the level of oxidant stress. All are in the form of simple statements that are easy to answer. You will see that even something that might appear benign to you has a biological influence. This test is obviously a broad indication and is no substitute for more advanced examinations from a healthcare practitioner. The scoring for the test follows the questions.

1. What is your body mass index (BMI)?

BMI is the ratio of your weight to your height. Your body mass is defined as your weight in kilograms (kg) divided by your height in meters (m) squared. For example, if you weigh 75 kg and measure 1.83 m in height, your body mass is 22.4—75 ÷ (1.83 x 1.83) = 22.4 BMI.

To convert to pounds and inches, multiply your weight in pounds by 704. Then multiply your height in inches by itself. Divide the first answer by the second answer for your BMI. For example, 165 pounds multiplied by 704 equals 116,160; a height of 6 feet is 72 inches, which multiplied by itself equals 5,184; 116,160 ÷ 5,184 = 22.4 BMI. You are allowed to use a calculator!

    A. Less than 18 or more than 30

    B. 18 or between 25 and 30

    C. Between 19 and 24

2. Check your blood pressure. (If you don't know your blood pressure, there is a good chance that it is normal, but do think about getting checked.) In which range do you fall?

    A. Above 150/95

    B. Between 150/95 and 140/90

    C. Between 140/90 and 120/80

    D. Below 120/80

3. Which of the following statements best characterizes your eating habits?

    A. I put emphasis on quality food and balanced meals.

    B. I regularly stray from a healthy diet.

    C. I adore fast food and eat few green vegetables.

4. How many meals do you eat each day?

    A. Three proper meals a day: breakfast, lunch, and dinner, and sometimes an afternoon snack

    B. One proper meal in the evening, no breakfast, snacks throughout the day

    C. Two proper meals, morning and evening, and lunch on the run

5. How often do you eat fruit and vegetables?

    A. Two or three times a week only

    B. Once a day

    C. Several times a day

It is interesting that the budget for promoting fruit and vegetables in the United States is $1 million.

For the same period, the budget of one of the leading fast-food companies is $800 million.

The result is that more than one in two Americans never eat fruit or vegetables.

Eighty million Americans are overweight compared to 5 million in France and 2 million in Japan.

6. How do you like your meat?

    A. Very well done

    B. Medium

    C. Rare

7. How do you like your french fries?

    A. Very crunchy

    B. Fairly crunchy

    C. Lightly golden

8. What sort of fish do you like?

   A. Fairly oily (salmon, tuna, sardines)

   B. Smoked

   C. Other categories

9. How often do you eat sweets and sugary cakes and cookies?

   A. A lot

   B. An average amount

   C. Never

10. What is your waist measurement?

   For men:
   A. More than 41.34 inches (105 cm)

   B. Between 37.4 and 41.34 inches (95 and 105 cm)

   C. Below 37.4 inches (95 cm)

   For women:
   A. More than 31.5 inches (80 cm)

   B. Between 27.56 and 31.5 inches (70 and 80 cm)

   C. Below 27.56 inches (70 cm)

11. Since the age of twenty, how much weight have you put on?

   A. More than 22 pounds (10 kilos)

   B. Between 11 and 22 pounds (5 and 10 kilos)

   C. Less than 11 pounds (5 kilos)

12. How much water (including herbal teas and infusions or natural juice) do you drink each day?

  A. 1.5 to 2.5 quarts (approximately 6 to 11 glasses)

  B. 1 to 1.5 quarts (approximately 4 to 6 glasses)

  C. Less than 1 quart (less than 4 glasses)

13. Are you in the habit of drinking alcohol?
(1 glass of wine = 2 beers; 1 aperitif = 2 glasses of wine)

  A. Several glasses of wine a day and strong alcohol regularly

  B. 2 or 3 glasses of wine a day and no strong alcohol

  C. Less than 1 glass of wine a day

  D. Never

14. Do you smoke?

  A. Yes

  B. I have never smoked

  C. I stopped recently

15. How many cigarettes do you smoke each day?
(1 average cigar = 3 cigarettes; 1 pipe = 5 cigarettes)

  A. Less than 10 cigarettes a day

  B. 1 cigarette from time to time

  C. More than 10 cigarettes a day

  D. I don't smoke

16. How many hours do you sleep each night?

   A. Between 7 and 9 hours

   B. Between 5 and 7 hours

   C. No more than 5 hours, feeling tired upon waking

17. How many hours of exercise do you get each week?

   A. More than 5 hours

   B. Between 3 and 5 hours

   C. Between 1 and 3 hours

   D. None

18. What is your attitude toward the sun?

   A. In summer, I sunbathe for several hours at a time, often without protection; in winter, I go for regular suntanning sessions.

   B. I use protection and try not to stay in the sun for too long.

19. What do you think of your wrinkles?

   A. They don't bother me.

   B. I can no longer bear to look in the mirror.

   C. I have gone in for treatment (injections, surgery).

20. How would you describe your feelings on your romantic life?

   A. I am happy in love.

   B. I am alone but that suits me.

   C. I am alone and wish I wasn't.

21. How often do you have sex?

    A. Three or four times a week

    B. Two or three times a month

    C. Never

22. Are you

    A. Often tense?

    B. Generally relaxed?

    C. Very calm and nearly always relaxed?

23. How would you describe your life?

    A. My life is satisfactory overall.

    B. Certain things could be better.

    C. My life is rather unsatisfactory; I would like many things to be different.

24. Does your work

    A. Bring satisfaction and pleasure even if you are sometimes under stress?

    B. Seem routine to you?

    C. Bring no satisfaction and demand too much of you?

25. Does your work take place in a polluted environment or have you run risks of professional intoxication?

    A. Yes

    B. No

    C. I don't know

26. In your family, have there been cases of cardiovascular illness, cancer, diabetes, or senile dementia?

    A. Many cases

    B. Several

    C. One or two

    D. None

27. Do you have parents or grandparents who have lived beyond the age of seventy-five?

    A. No

    B. Yes, one

    C. Yes, two

    D. Yes, more than two

28. Where do you live?

    A. In a city

    B. In the country

    C. In a city and the country, alternately

29. After eating, do you suffer from any of the following symptoms? (Circle all that apply.)

    A. Itching

    B. Headaches

    C. Flatulence

    D. Runny nose

    E. Nothing

30. Do you take antioxidants?

    A. Yes, regularly

    B. Yes, from time to time

    C. Never

31. Are you familiar with the CRP (C-reactive protein) test?

    A. Yes, and I know my results.

    B. I have heard about it.

    C. I've never heard of it.

32. Do you take omega-3s?

    A. Yes, between 2 and 3 grams per day

    B. Yes, less than 1 gram per day

    C. Never

33. Are you

    A. Always in a hurry?

    B. Busy but you take time to do things?

    C. Never in a hurry?

See next page for test-scoring results.

TEST SCORING

For each question, find the corresponding number of points for your answer. Then, add up the total to discover your aptitude for staying young.

1. **A.** 1 point **B.** 2 points **C.** 3 points

2. **A.** 0 points **B.** 2 points **C.** 3 points **D.** 1 point

3. **A.** 3 points **B.** 2 points **C.** 1 point

4. **A.** 3 points **B.** 1 point **C.** 2 points

5. **A.** 1 point **B.** 2 points **C.** 3 points

6. **A.** 1 point **B.** 2 points **C.** 3 points

7. **A.** 1 point **B.** 2 points **C.** 3 points

8. **A.** 3 points **B.** 1 point **C.** 2 points

9. **A.** 1 point **B.** 2 points **C.** 3 points

10. **A.** −1 point **B.** 0 points **C.** 1 point

11. **A.** 0 points **B.** 1 point **C.** 3 points

12. **A.** 3 points **B.** 2 points **C.** 1 point

13. **A.** −1 point **B.** 1 point **C.** 3 points **D.** 4 points

14. **A.** −1 point **B.** 4 points **C.** 0 points

15. **A.** 0 points **B.** 1 point **C.** −1 point **D.** 4 points

16. **A.** 3 points **B.** 2 points **C.** 1 point

17. **A.** 3 points **B.** 2 points **C.** 1 point **D.** 0 points

18. **A.** 1 point **B.** 3 points

19. **A.** 2 points **B.** 0 points **C.** 1 point

20. **A.** 3 points **B.** 2 points **C.** 1 point

21. **A.** 4 points **B.** 2 points **C.** 0 points

22. **A.** 1 point **B.** 2 points **C.** 3 points

23. **A.** 3 points **B.** 2 points **C.** 0 points

24. **A.** 3 points **B.** 2 points **C.** 1 point

25. **A.** −2 points **B.** 1 point **C.** 0 points

26.	**A.** 0 points	**B.** 1 point	**C.** 2 points	**D.** 3 points	
27.	**A.** 0 points	**B.** 1 point	**C.** 2 points	**D.** 3 points	
28.	**A.** −1 point	**B.** 2 points	**C.** 1 point		
29.	**A.** −1 point	**B.** −1 point	**C.** −1 point	**D.** −1 point	**E.** 2 points
30.	**A.** 3 points	**B.** 2 points	**C.** 1 point		
31.	**A.** 3 points	**B.** 2 points	**C.** 1 point		
32.	**A.** 3 points	**B.** 2 points	**C.** 1 point		
33.	**A.** −1 point	**B.** 1 point	**C.** 2 points		

ANALYSIS OF RESULTS

- **More than 70 points—Excellent aptitude for staying young.** Your biological and apparent age is certainly inferior to your chronological age. You appear up to seven years younger than your age, and that's great. Continue to take care of yourself to maintain your balance and make your health capital prosper even more.

- **Between 50 and 70 points—Good aptitude for staying young.** Your biological age (your age based on the condition of your body) corresponds more or less to your chronological age. Don't forget: it is better to take precautions than to grow old. Change your bad habits by following the advice in this book and you will increase your vital capital.

- **Less than 50 points—Weak aptitude for staying young.** An accelerated aging process is lying in wait for you. Your biological age is definitely greater than your chronological age. You might look up to seven years older than your age, unfortunately. It's up to you to take action: change your lifestyle immediately to turn the corner as quickly as possible and safeguard your vitality. Also, see your doctor immediately, because it is better to take precautions than it is to grow old prematurely.

Remember: this test is only intended as a guide. In no way does it replace full medical tests and examinations.

CHAPTER 1

Getting Started

et me introduce Julien, one of my patients. He is a very smart young man who works for an advertising company and likes to enjoy his life. When we start our conversation, he does not believe in preventive medicine for aging.

JULIEN: *I'm thirty-eight years old—what has a book on aging got to do with me?*

DR. CHAUCHARD: This book is not just for elderly people; it is for all those who want to live in full health for as long as possible. For older readers, it will be a case of learning to age in the best way. But adults of all ages should be concerned because we start growing old not just after the age of fifty but from the moment we are born. In our society, we have not yet grasped this revolutionary understanding of the body, let alone allowed it to affect the way we live our lives.

Showing you how to live for a long time is just one of the objectives of this book. In addition to adding years to your life, you can also add life to your years. In short, you can rejuvenate yourself with this program! Youth passes swiftly, marked by growth spurts. As Paul Nizan wrote at the start of his famous book *Aden Arabie,* "I was twenty years old. I wouldn't let anyone say that it's the best time of your life." At the other extreme, old age fades away, and our life with it. What remains, in the middle, is a period of undetermined length that we call the age of maturity—adult life—which is also the active life, the time for seeking fulfillment in our work and our love life.

How many years does the age of adult maturity last?

Some people retire at age sixty, others are still working at the highest level when they are seventy-five years old. We can all think of an example of someone who is "old before his time" as the expression goes, and, at the other extreme, a person who seems forty-something but is actually sixty-five. The age of maturity is the only period of life that can vary from one individual to another. Everyone then declines at differing speeds, with varying degrees of success. We wonder how the French actor Jean Gabin who played in *Grand Illusion* (1937) could have become the old man in *The Cat* (1971). In this case, we succumb to the "grand illusion" that someone could remain the pinup of French cinema all his life, whether he was thirty or sixty-five. It's the same problem today for those who let the time pass without seizing it and holding it back—without controlling that which is most precious to us, life and the quality of life.

I don't want to pay attention to everything I'm doing. I want to take advantage of my life, accept that what will happen will happen. That is my first choice, so what do you say to that?

Today, looking old is a choice—it is no longer an obligation. Of course, almost everyone knows that, and it's nothing new. People generally say, "I'm prepared," or "I'm taking care of myself," or "I'm looking after my body." But how much are they, really? If that is your choice, to not pay attention to your health, enjoy it—but bear in mind that you are exposing yourself to an accelerated aging process.

Of course, I'm careful about what I eat. I haven't played team sports since I left school, but I belong to the local gym. I even went on a spa cure vacation to the Mediterranean last summer. I lost at least six pounds—not bad—and I was incredibly fit for a month. But once I was back at work and under stress, the weight went straight back on.

Our lives resemble Balzac's "skin of sorrow": a piece of leather that shrinks and shrinks with every day. We have always burned the candle at both ends and are starting to pay the price. After the age of twenty-five, we are increasingly prone to the blues—we tell ourselves it's normal, that everyone goes through these slight depressions, that it will disappear as quickly as it came. One day, it's sexual failure, followed by almost total disappearance of erections that have become more and more difficult. It's the arteries, says the doctor, they are less supple. Or it's diabetes or high cholesterol or high blood pressure or prostate problems. Then other problems start to creep up on us: hearing and sight problems, kidney insufficiency, arthritis, maybe even a nervous breakdown, and, very often, a weight problem. Whatever our issues, they paint an engrossing picture.

We are not all good or all bad—we age little by little. But is it still the fate of people, in this new century, to die "in detail" as Voltaire said, in little detached pieces, organs and functions dying one after the other?

No, absolutely not. It is true that I want to "live for a long time"
certainly, but not to "live like an old man" . . .

It is, firstly, a social and economic reality: studying and training last longer and longer, so we are starting our working lives later. How many CEOs are under forty years old? And, of course, a lawyer at forty-five years of age, who has been practicing the law for several years, is more experienced than a twenty-five-year-old novice. But the value of experience is a double-edged sword: there is no point in being experienced if the body is beginning to fail. This is equally true in our professional and our sex lives. It is a sad fact that a soccer player can only kick a ball hard until the age of thirty, barely enough time to make all the mistakes that teach him his job—a job that, thanks to its physical nature, he or she will soon only be able to exercise from the sidelines. Society and businesses need young men and women—with experience. It's a contradiction in terms, but nevertheless the ideal résumé. Every advertisement for a senior executive mentions "experience required." The ideal profile for a manager combines physical and psychological health—in other words, youth and experience, therefore, maturity.

All the same, French president Jacques Chirac is over seventy years old . . .

Yes, but a fuss was made recently about Jacques Chirac's hearing problems, which are very common in a man of seventy-one years. "It is absurd," retort Chirac's supporters, "everyone can see he is in excellent health." Certainly the president, hale and hearty with no white hair and still attractive, doesn't look his age. He appears to be in perfect health. Even so, the physical condition of the president is always microscopically examined and Mr. Chirac, like everyone else, has no wish to be labelled "old." Look at film actor and director Clint Eastwood—he just won an Academy Award for directing *Million Dollar Baby* at the age of seventy-four!

The modern active person, regardless of his or her age, needs physical energy to travel, attend meetings, go to business lunches, read through reports—to do the 1,001 things required to keep the show on the road. He or she must cope with travel fatigue and jet lag. Add in the demands of a family and you will see our manager doesn't often get to rest. Many of us have to think of everything and never stop—we are obliged to have the stamina of a twenty-year-old.

"Looking young" is the watchword—fashionable neckties and a cool way of speaking. In contrast, the value of "old" is in decline. Listen to how we talk: "looks old," "he's aged," "old bloke," "old hat," "old maid." The notion of old age is pejorative today. "Old" is a word that every person wishes to strike out of the dictionary and one that we don't hesitate to hurl at our worst enemy when we want to reinforce an insult: "The old b———!"

What age can we hope to live to?

Here, we're talking about biological reality. This is as paradoxical as youthful maturity. The human potential for life is 120 years, but man lives in a regressive state from the age of twenty-five! Don't believe that this life expectancy of more than a century is mere science fiction: there are already plenty of people who are 100 years old. This potential life expectancy of 120 years is recognized by all specialists in the genetic theory of aging and is based on the life expectancy of the chromosomes. Between 1900 and 1950, life expectancy increased by four or five years. Now that we are having greater success in controlling the pathologies related to excess weight and atherosclerosis, and in preventing the development of cancer by bringing in effective treatments, our life expectancy has increased by even more. One child out of two born today has a life expectancy of 100 years. We can, therefore, now consider without any exaggeration that a man or woman of forty or fifty years is only halfway through his or her potential life. Unfortunately, too often, on the physical and psychological front, the person is more than halfway through his or her actual life.

Why?

Above all, because we generally don't take care of ourselves as we get older.

It is in human nature to deteriorate physically. It is not "natural" to worry about one's health too soon, to start preventive treatments at the age of twenty-five . . .

Yet that is what young people are already doing in other countries. I am thinking especially of Japan.

Even so, I am not going to start taking anti-wrinkle pills when I've only just finished using products for younger skin! I've got all the time in the world to go for check-ups and take medicine.

This recklessness is puerile and regrettable but is rooted in our mentality and in the way we live: this facility for procrastination is not always as noble and profound as that of Hamlet. The "wait until later" approach is the real cause of our future deficiencies.

I want to try to age less quickly, but I don't want to change the way I live.

We all want to learn individually to control our advance into old age. Therefore, we must give ourselves the means to do so. Today, we have the power to insure our physical condition the way we insure our home. We just need to seek out the insurer, your anti-aging specialist. He will detect for you the main risk factors and define for you the policy for a better lifestyle.

All that would be much too complicated for me. I was useless at biology in school.

My proposal is not that of a biology teacher, and you are not a medical student. Obviously, all this theory interests me, but what *you* are really interested in is your well-being. My objective is very concrete, very practical: in reading this book, you will get a precise idea about the phenomena associated with aging and the treatments that exist today, and by becoming aware of the medical revolution going on, you will not bypass things that can change your life for the better.

What are the risks if I do nothing?

Many people—and it's deplorable—do not notice that they are aging before they hit fifty. It is what I call the "big change." But this kind of change, frankly, one could do without! So as not to create too much anxiety for those reading this, I prefer to enumerate the signs of the "big change" without too much detail. Study closely the following lists that summarize the signs of "male menopause" (andropause) and female menopause, the two great problems of advancing age, and you will see that they are similar.

Alright, if I want to fight against aging, what are the successive stages that will allow me to live better for longer and to regain control of my health?

Nothing can be clearly established unless you and your doctor evaluate your biological strengths and weaknesses, both physical and psychological. This is because the most important thing of all, as Socrates used to say, is to know yourself.

When should I start the program?

Now! I prefer to insist on the notion of "age-preventive medicine" rather than "anti-aging medicine," which is the term used more often in the United States. I recommend and encourage prevention: it is never too late or too early to start. Prevention is better than cure.

SYMPTOMS OF ANDROPAUSE ("MALE CHANGE OF LIFE")

VASOMOTOR

- hot flushes
- cold limbs
- sweating
- palpitations
- racing pulse
- headaches

PSYCHOLOGICAL

- nervousness
- irritability
- insomnia
- depression
- negative self-image
- antisocial tendencies
- feeling like crying
- suicidal tendencies
- pins and needles, skin prickling
- inability to concentrate

CONSTITUTIONAL

- weakness
- fatigue
- muscular pain
- painful joints
- loss of appetite
- nausea and vomiting
- constipation
- weight loss

URINARY

- diminished stream of urine
- frequent need to urinate
- difficulties in urinating

SEXUAL

- diminished libido
- difficult erections

Does it require a lot of effort?

We must start at the beginning and the beginning requires courage. You can stop when you want. You are free to follow me in my challenge or to stop when it seems right to you.

SYMPTOMS OF MENOPAUSE ("FEMALE CHANGE OF LIFE")

VASOMOTOR

- hot flushes
- dizziness
- cold extremities
- sweating
- palpitations
- racing pulse
- headaches

PSYCHOLOGICAL

- sleep problems
- nervousness
- excitability
- irritability
- depression
- negative self-image
- antisocial tendencies
- feeling like crying
- suicidal tendencies
- pins and needles, skin prickling
- difficulty concentrating

CONSTITUTIONAL

- weakness
- fatigue

- constipation
- diminished vision
- painful joints
- increased appetite
- nausea and vomiting
- stomachaches
- diffused pain
- weight gain

URINARY

- loss of strength in urine stream
- repeated cystitis
- frequent desire to urinate
- difficulty urinating

SEXUAL

- decreased libido
- less vaginal lubrication
- irregular sexual relations

MENSTRUAL

- irregular menstrual cycle
- lighter periods
- cessation of menstruation

Where must I start?

Drink less, smoke less, eat less sugar and less salt. All these things considerably increase the risks associated with aging and often reduce the efficiency of programs geared to fight the phenomena linked to aging. "Smoking kills" is written on your cigarette packs and in books on medicine, so you have been warned. But eating badly also kills. It's not yet written on any packaging, but we can expect a real reaction against fast food and junk food. We need to register our changing attitudes, our changing tastes, our rejection of that which is too sweet, too fatty, overcooked, and not organic, our rejection of soft drinks and the return to good fruit juice that we squeeze ourselves. What happened to cigarette manufacturers ten years ago could well happen to certain fast-food giants.

For now, I am merely sounding an alarm bell. But as a doctor concerned with good nutrition, my duty is to point the finger at major excess. Here's an example: if you eat in a good restaurant with good butter, you will absorb only 8 grams of fat, whereas at the same moment your child may eat a fast-food hamburger and absorb 33 grams of fat. And that's not all: the cooked saturated fats present in fast food do the maximum damage to cells and their membranes. We are therefore pushing our children into "bad eating" and "bad living" by allowing them to eat fast food. This is not to mention the excess of sugar in cakes and sweet drinks. The overconsumption of fast food and junk food is very serious and we need to do something now.

CHAPTER 2

Inflammation Causes Aging

JULIEN: *I'm beginning to realize what is waiting for me if I do nothing. I'd better watch out . . .*

DR. CHAUCHARD: Good! An aware patient who is watching out is a patient half cured!

Where must I start if I want to understand and control my aging?

Start at the beginning, of course, and inflammation of the cell membranes is one of the primary causes of aging. It is the most important phenomenon and yet the least understood in the theory of aging. Cell membranes suffer and age more quickly because of inflammation. They are covered with (among other things) hormone receptors and neurotransmitters, which permit our bodies to function. Because hormones and neurotransmitters can affect every part of the body, these inflammatory reactions are considered to play a part in numerous pathologies related to the aging process.

What is inflammation?

If you've ever twisted your ankle, you've experienced inflammation. The inflammation syndrome, in its acute form, is marked by three symptoms: redness, pain, and heat. The ankle gets larger and swells up due to the action of cell secretions called cytokines. The cells also produce substances to repair the damage done at the site of the lesion, causing a vasodilation (a dilation of the blood vessels), which causes redness and heat.

This inflammation process at the cellular level provokes the destruction of intra-membrane fatty acids, which brings about a series of chain reactions through the guidance of the cytokines and leads to the formation of free radicals. Free radicals are reactive molecules that cause damage in the body.

As we get older, free-radical damage accumulates and, little by little, rigidifies the cell membranes, making them less fluid and less permeable, and the receptors on the surface that receive hormones, nutrients, proteins, amino acids, and minerals are damaged. The trans-membrane passage (via the membrane) of fatty acids is then disrupted. Not only is the cell badly nourished, but the infiltration of free radicals is then considerable, enabling them to reach the center of the cell (in other words, the nucleus) and in turn to alter our genetic code. The cell can no longer reproduce itself identically—this then accelerates the rate of aging.

Inflammation and, hence, free-radical damage, can be caused by something physical, such as heat, cold, or ionizing radiation, or result from exposure to chemical substances, notably acid or basic compositions or bacterial toxins. It can also be provoked by an immune reaction, the consequence of an infection with pathogenic organisms like bacteria, viruses, parasites, or fungi.

How do we measure an inflammatory reaction?

C-reactive protein is secreted by the liver. It is an essential player in inflammation and by measuring it in a blood test we can obtain a good evaluation of the inflammatory activity that is affecting the organism.

What are the consequences of inflammatory reactions?

We have enumerated the damage at the microscopic level. On the scale of the human body, inflammation plays a role in a large number of pathological conditions, including anemia, allergies, cardiovascular and neurodegenerative illnesses, strokes, and pathologies relating to the joints.

Inflammation is everywhere in our bodies, and in the brain it is manifested in degenerative illnesses like Parkinson's disease and Alzheimer's disease. In the joints, it is called rheumatism, arthritis, and permanent joint pain. In the heart, inflammation causes angina and myocardial infarction (heart attack). In the bones, it is osteoporosis and deformation. And in the skin, we see it as wrinkles and dehydration, dull complexion, and problem texture.

How can we fight this enemy that is inflammation?

If we adopt better anti-inflammatory eating habits and take an excellent multivitamin and mineral supplement, we can do a lot. With the simple blood test for C-reactive protein, we can anticipate the reactions of our organism and so measure the speed with which we are repairing our cell membranes. For that, we must not forget a good breakfast—as I describe it in my program—and we must eat plenty of protein, especially oily fish.

What is the link between inflammation and cardiovascular illness?

The most immediate danger of chronic inflammation is that it makes the atheroma plates along the arteries more vulnerable to rupturing. When an atheroma plate breaks, it liberates pieces of tissue that can settle in the arteries nourishing the cardiac muscle or in the vessels that supply oxygen to the brain cells. The final result can be an infarction or stroke when the blood vessels break or are obstructed. There now exists convincing proof that inflammation is strongly linked to heart attacks and strokes.

What is the effect of inflammation on the brain and what can be done?

It has recently been recognized that inflammation plays a central role in the debilitating cognitive decline that characterizes neurological troubles such as Alzheimer's disease or vascular dementia. Although mental decline and loss of memory have until now been considered inevitable characteristics of old age, new research suggests that such inflammation and age-associated decline could be prevented. This could signify that, to a certain degree, neuro-inflammation is nothing other than incidental to old age. Therefore, controlling the inflammation could help prevent subsequent memory loss or cognitive decline.

How can we combat these inflammatory reactions?

In a general manner, one way of fighting inflammation, and relieving the pain it causes, is to stop the secretions of the inflammatory cells, the cytokines. Therefore, we need to lessen their activity.

People in good health but with high levels of C-reactive protein must try to bring this down with anti-inflammatory substances: tocopherols (vitamin E), borage oil (rich in omega-6 fatty acids), fish oils (rich in omega-3 fatty acids), and the hormone DHEA (dehydroepiandrosterone). Two new products, GliSODin (superoxide dismutase) and Lyprinol (the extract of the green-lipped mussel *Perna canaliculus*), are very effective.

To produce a significant result, it is necessary to take at least 3–4 grams per day of omega-3s and 1 gram per day of omega-6s (both polyunsaturated fatty acids). A study conducted on subjects suffering from rheumatic diseases shows that fish oil lowers the concentration of dangerous cytokines by up to 90 percent. Olive oil is also very effective— it requires at least 2–3 tablespoons a day to feel the benefit, but it really does work.

You will find all these anti-inflammatory substances in the nutritional program that I reveal later in the book.

CHAPTER 3

A Four-Day Trial

JULIEN: *Why is our diet, as well as our digestion, so important?*

DR. CHAUCHARD: The intestine is a second brain: It produces at least twenty neurotransmitters, including serotonin, which governs our mood, appetite, and sleep patterns. The surface area of the villi could cover a tennis court. The intestine contains 10,000 billion bacteria. Mucus controls its permeability. The lymph tissue is 80 percent balanced by the intestinal tissue, which absorbs 60,000 pounds of food and nearly 40,000 gallons of water during its lifetime. Recognizing the central role of the intestine helps us to better understand the importance of drinking water and the value of nutrition in a healthy life.

I think I am now motivated to start eating better. How can I start? Isn't it too soon? Is the program difficult to follow?

I suggest that you start by eating differently for four days in order to appear four years younger. Try the following program—it is simple and effective, provided that you are serious about it. You can then test my inflammatory theory of cellular aging, which you are in the process of discovering, for yourself.

For four days, you will cut out all inflammatory foods and strengthen your diet with antioxidants (to fight free radicals), in addition to omega-3 and omega-6 fatty acids. After four days, be objective: look at your complexion, your wrinkles, test your mood, your sense of vitality, and appreciate your rejuvenation, because it has just begun.

EAT BETTER, EAT DIFFERENTLY: THE GOLDEN RULES

Use the following eight rules as your guide through the four-day trial.

1. Proteins first—start every meal with protein.

2. Drink more water. Here is a formula* to determine the appropriate amount of water (in liters) to keep your body healthy: add your height in centimeters plus your weight in kilograms, then divide by 100. For example, if you measure 1.70 meters high and weigh 70 kilograms, it will be $(170 + 70) \div 100 = 2.4$ liters of water per day, every day (and more when the weather is hot). Drink a glass of water roughly every hour.

3. Eat three meals a day, plus a snack (an oily vegetable and sugar from fruit) between 4 P.M. and 5 P.M.; the natural peak of insulin occurs at this time of day, which is favorable to the absorption of sugar.

4. Stay away from the foods that dramatically stimulate the pancreas and provoke excessive insulin secretions, such as coffee, fast food, and sugary foods (see "Foods to Avoid" in Chapter 10).

5. When you get up in the morning, immediately drink a glass of water (room temperature) and do the same before eating breakfast. Coffee is not allowed, as it is inflammatory—coffee stimulates the secretion of insulin and cortisol.

6. Every hour after your breakfast, drink a glass of water or a cup of tea (green or other tea). You can add lemon zest to your water if you like. You can also add chlorophyll to the water and mint to the tea.

7. Normally, you should urinate at around 11 A.M. and 12:30 P.M., and then 3 P.M., 5 P.M., 7 P.M., 9 P.M., and once during the night, for a total of seven times in twenty-four hours (at least).

---

*Metric measurements are required for this formula. A conversion chart can help you figure your height in centimeters and weight in kilograms, if necessary.

8. If you are hungry, eat more proteins or increase the quantity of olive oil (extra-virgin, first cold-pressing).

FIRST EVENING

Begin your four-day trial the night before day one (we will end with lunch on day four). To give yourself a reference point, start by weighing yourself and measuring your chest, waist, hips, and thighs. Then between 7 P.M. and 8 P.M., eat the following:

- 8.75–10.5 ounces of baked salmon plus olive oil and lemon juice. Look for salmon from Alaska because it is always wild (farming salmon is forbidden in Alaska). It is very rich in omega-3 fatty acids. Failing this, choose organic or other good-quality salmon. For those who don't like salmon, it can be replaced by tuna or another oily fish (mackerel, red mullet, John Dory, sardines, fresh herring, unsalted fresh anchovies, trout, Atlantic halibut, swordfish, pink trout, eel).

- 1 cup of endive or other allowed vegetables, including all forms of lettuce, asparagus, broccoli, Brussels sprouts, cauliflower, celery, cucumber, cabbage (green, red, or Chinese), green or yellow beans, mushrooms, onions, spinach, summer squash, sweet and hot peppers, tomatoes, and zucchini. Add olive oil to taste.

FIRST DAY

Begin day one by drinking a large glass of water (room temperature) upon waking. Have another glass of water or a cup of tea before breakfast. Then, eat according to the following menus.

Breakfast

- 6.25 ounces of salmon (not smoked) plus olive oil and lemon juice

- 2–3 ounces of whole-grain bread (not white bread) plus olive oil

- 2–3 ounces of cheese (blue cheese, brie, cottage cheese, feta, goat's cheese, full- or low-fat mozzarella, Muenster, parmesan, Romano,

Roquefort). If you don't like cheese, replace it with olive oil, unsalted butter, or avocado.

- Tea, water, or an herbal infusion. Don't add any sugar or artificial sweeteners.

Lunch

- 7–8.75 ounces of salmon or tuna (large morsels)

- 7–8.75 ounces of green vegetables and/or broccoli

- 1 or 2 servings of Salad Nicoise (see below)

Salad Nicoise

YIELD: TWO SERVINGS

2 hardboiled eggs

7 ounces of roast chicken

7 ounces of sardines in oil

2 tomatoes, sliced

10 green and black olives

3.5 ounces of cooked green beans

1 tablespoon of chopped basil

1 tablespoon of thyme

1 teaspoon of oregano, olive oil, and balsamic vinegar mixture

Cut the eggs and the chicken into small pieces, crumble the sardines, and then gently mix all the ingredients together.

4 P.M. Snack

- 6.25 ounces of chicken or turkey breast, or 1 avocado with olive oil and lemon juice, or 2 small squares of dark chocolate (with at least 70 percent cocoa content, not milk chocolate). It is easy to carry around some dark chocolate or an apple—everyone can do that, at the office or elsewhere—for a healthy snack.

- 1 grapefruit or other fruit (apple, apricot, cherries, berries, other citrus fruit such as an orange, melon other than watermelon, peach, pear, persimmon, plum, rhubarb)

Dinner

- At least 8.75 ounces of tuna or mackerel, with onions, tomatoes, olive oil, and lemon juice

- 1 cup of steamed spinach plus olive oil

SECOND DAY

Begin day two by drinking a large glass of water (room temperature) upon waking. Have another glass of water or a cup of tea before breakfast. Then, eat according to the following menus.

Breakfast

- 3.5 ounces of chicken or turkey breast plus a little olive oil *or* an omelette made with 3 egg whites and 1 yolk plus a little olive oil

- 1.5–1.75 ounces of whole-grain bread (not white bread) plus olive oil

- 2–3 ounces of cheese (if you don't like cheese, choose a quality unsalted butter or spread your bread with olive oil)

Lunch

- 8.75 ounces of grilled salmon (remove any burnt bits, as anything too well grilled is high in inflammatory and carcinogenic substances) plus olive oil and lemon juice

- 1 cup of green beans (steamed) plus olive oil

- 1.75 ounces of whole-grain bread (not white bread) plus olive oil; or a little brown rice or whole-wheat pasta (1 small bowl)

4 P.M. Snack

- 2 squares of dark chocolate (minimum 70 percent cocoa content)

- 1 apple

Dinner

A practical piece of advice: have dinner half an hour earlier than usual tonight. Moving up your bedtime by half an hour tonight is another excellent idea.

- 8.75 ounces of salmon with aniseed

- 1 cup of endive or other approved vegetable (see list under "First Evening" on page 35)

THIRD DAY

Begin day three by drinking a large glass of water (room temperature) upon waking. Have another glass of water or a cup of tea before breakfast. Then, eat according to the following menus.

Breakfast

- 3.5 ounces of grilled salmon plus olive oil and 1 slice of lemon

- 2–3 ounces of whole-grain bread (not white bread) plus olive oil

- 2–3 ounces of cheese (if you don't like cheese, choose a quality unsalted butter or spread your bread with olive oil)

Lunch

- At least 8.75 ounces of tuna, roasted in the oven with 1 cup of chopped tomatoes and onions

- 1 serving of Salad Nicoise (see page 36)

- 1 small bowl of brown rice

4 P.M. Snack

- 1 avocado plus olive oil or 2 squares of dark chocolate (minimum 70 percent cocoa)
- 10–15 raspberries, blackberries, or other red fruit

Dinner

- 8.75 ounces of salmon plus olive oil and lemon juice
- 1 cup of broccoli (steamed)

One hour before going to bed, eat 3 almonds.

FOURTH DAY

Begin day four by drinking a large glass of water (room temperature) upon waking. Have another glass of water or a cup of tea before breakfast. Then, eat according to the following menus.

Breakfast

- An omelette made with 3 egg whites and 1 yolk (or 2 yolks if you have low cholesterol)
- 3.5 ounces of chilled salmon
- 2 slices of cantaloupe or melon

Lunch

- 7–8.75 ounces salmon or tuna (large morsels)
- 1–2 cups of chicory or spinach
- 1 serving of Salad Nicoise (see page 36)

Don't forget your afternoon snack, and finish your day with a light dinner including the fish of your choice and vegetables.

THE RESULTS

Congratulations! Your trial program is finished. Judge the results for yourself.

- Palm of the hand test—Press the two interior muscles, the thumb muscle and the one facing it: these two muscles will be firmer. We call these muscular centers the thenar and hypothenar loges. The trial program stops insulin secretions as much as possible to reduce the secretion of aldehydes and cytokines. These chemicals are doing some damage in the cell membranes. When the damage stops, you will immediately see the skin becoming better and shinier.

- Take stock of your muscular pain—I am sure that it will be reduced.

- Look at your hairbrush—There are probably fewer than ten hairs attached to it today. The program makes intestinal absorption more effective and accurate, so that iron and amino acid absorption is optimized. Consequently, your hair and scalp metabolism are improved.

- Weigh yourself—You will certainly have lost some weight over the four days, probably between two and four pounds.

- Check your complexion, your wrinkles, and the whites of your eyes—You will see the difference.

I hope you are now convinced that this program can help you look and feel younger and rejuvenated. We will now look at other reasons why this method is so effective and then outline the full program later in the book.

CHAPTER 4

Controlling Insulin
to Stay Slim

JULIEN: *I've decided to stop smoking and drink less alcohol. What should I attack next?*

DR. CHAUCHARD: You should now work toward controlling your body's secretion of the hormone insulin, as high levels are linked to excess weight, which is in turn connected to aging. Being overweight is the number-one enemy of vitality.

Is the problem the same for men and women?

Body fat is distributed differently in men and women. Men accumulate fat in the upper part of the body (an apple shape) and women in the lower part (a pear shape). Another difference is the inequality in the risks linked to obesity. In men, obesity brings increased frequency in diabetes, coronary illness, and premature death, whereas women are relatively well protected until menopause.

How can you explain this correlation between being overweight and getting old?

In 1999, Dr. Thomas Perls, a Harvard researcher who had been conducting studies on more than 100 people aged around 100, released some interesting information about their eating patterns. On a nutritional level, the only common denominator among these 100-year-olds was that they had eaten frugally throughout their lives. Only 1 percent of them had ever been overweight. Do you know many people who are overweight, diabetic, overstressed, and over 100 years old? No, of course not, and neither do I; I don't know any.

As we get older, we have a natural tendency to get fatter. We can't just chalk this phenomenon up to overindulgent business lunches. We should look instead at the effect of insulin on our cell receptors.

What is the role of insulin in this phenomenon?

Insulin is a hormone that opens the receptors of the cell, the go-between that allows sugar to enter into the cell so that it can be transformed into energy. With age, in 75 percent of the population, the cell membrane surface becomes less sensitive to the action of insulin: the gate gets creaky and becomes more and more difficult to open, metaphorically speaking. This is the phenomenon known as "insulin resistance": insulin is secreted in normal quantities by a pancreas that is still working well, but the insulin is no longer capable of assuming its role at the level of its target organs—the muscles, the liver, and the adipose tissue.

Insulin plays an essential role in the storing of sugar and the production of energy within the cell. With insulin resistance, ever-larger amounts of the hormone are required to open the gate and transform the intracellular sugar into energetic substance. This tends to result in a higher rate of glycemia (glucose in the blood) and, consequently, a permanent stimulation of the pancreas, which makes excessive quantities of insulin. Rather as if you began by taking a little stick to kill a fly and then went on to use a hammer—you shouldn't be surprised by the hole in the table!

In a vicious circle, this excessive secretion of insulin—called hyperinsulinism—increases the desire for sugar and gives an impression of hunger; we, therefore, consume more and more sugar, which is less and less well stored by the cell. This sugar is then found in the blood and recovered by the liver, which transforms it not into energy but into fat. The trash can for fat is the bottom (especially in women) and the stomach (especially in men), and excess weight is only the tip of the iceberg.

The insulin-resistance phenomenon explains why, when we get to the age of fifty, we find found ourselves, on average, twenty pounds heavier than we were at age twenty (or even heavier if the insulin resistance is greater). The smaller percentage of people who do not put on weight are those who have low insulin secretion to begin with, in whom sugar is transformed into energy by the cell; they, therefore, are not victims of insulin resistance.

But the most destructive effect takes place at the cellular level. Hyperinsulinism is not constant—it is characterized by attacks of secretion that damage the cell membranes in the manner of a flame-thrower. This is also an inflammatory reaction. These attacks are so acute that they provoke a chain reaction that results in the secretion of cytokines, the "serial killers" of cell membranes. The cytokines and their chemical derivatives disturb the structure of the membranes. This is microscopic damage that one cannot feel but that, repeated regularly in the long term, explains why certain people will age more quickly than others. The cell walls gradually weaken under the ramming action of the ravaging force of the insulin secretions, provoked by eating rapidly absorbed sugars or "bad carbohydrates." (See "Sources of Carbohydrates and Sugars to Avoid" on page 44.)

How can we fight effectively against excess weight and hyperinsulinism?

There is no single direct cause responsible for making people over-weight (excessive calorie intake, for example). Rather, excess weight is the result of a metabolic chain reaction that is rooted in the nature of the foods we choose:

1. Excess weight is the consequence of hyperinsulinism, which encourages the creation of fatty reserves.

2. Hyperinsulinism is, in turn, the consequence of hyperglycemia.

3. Hyperglycemia is itself the consequence of a glycemic level that is too high in a meal.

4. Finally, the glycemic level of a meal is the consequence of a too-high proportion in that meal of carbohydrates with a high glycemic index. (See "Choose Foods According to the Glycemic Index" on page 46.)

Fighting excess weight is, therefore, a question of containing insulin

SOURCES OF CARBOHYDRATES AND SUGARS TO AVOID

White flour—In all products containing enriched flour, bleached flour, unbleached flour, semolina flour, corn flour, pasta, pizza crust, bagels, pretzels, tortillas, rolls, and most breads and other baked foods.

White rice—In foods containing white rice and enriched rice, polished rice, and rice flour in the list of ingredients.

Sugar and sweeteners—In foods that contain the following: sugar barley, sugar beet, brown sugar, Demerara sugar, corn syrup, date syrup, dextrose, malt, fructose, fruit juice and concentrated fruit juice, glucose, honey, inverted sugar, lactose, malt syrup, maltose, maple syrup, maple sugar, raw sugar, and sucrose. The quick way to spot sweeteners on the label is to look for the word "sugar" in any form, especially in words ending in the suffix "-ose."

production. By acting on the glycemic parameters of food, we can vary the insulin response and consequently control our weight gain. We, therefore, need to learn not to eat less but to eat better and at appropriate times during the day. By controlling our diet and lifestyle, and by engaging in regular exercise, we can grow old while avoiding the risk of inflammation and hyperinsulinism.

Does the solution lie, as we hear everywhere, in restricting our calorie intake? How can we get away from the frustration and restriction of diets?

No, it's not a question of eating less but rather of eating better, which means eating well at the right moment. Tell me what you want to eat and I will tell you when you can eat it. This is a real revolution, more important than the one described by Dr. Robert Atkins more than ten years ago.

There is a big leap from spontaneous calorie restriction to voluntary restriction. In reality, if the calorie intake is already low, it seems to me neither easy nor desirable to lower the average intake of energy still further. Restricting calories imposes a daily hardship on those who do it because it involves being almost permanently hungry. Plus, it is a source of considerable deficits in micronutrients, deficits that must be filled up if we are not to fall into bad nutrition. It can be a particular threat to health at certain times of our life, such as childhood, during pregnancy, and as we grow older. Finally, scientific research tells us that 95 percent of people who lose weight put it back on in a short period of time.

So, in view of all this, is there a reliable solution to the problem of excess weight? Nutrition must extend to an eating pattern that is harmonized to suit the individual, who must eat according to his or her personal tastes and individual metabolic capacities, and, above all, at the right time of day.

Eating less is therefore not a recommended strategy for living longer. On the other hand, we can reap the benefits of eating better and avoid becoming overweight by limiting recreational foods, especially those that provoke a dramatic rise in our blood sugar level (sweets, chocolate bars, soft drinks, white bread eaten between meals, and so on).

What diet or eating pattern do you recommend to avoid the insulin-resistance phenomenon?

I have good news and bad news. The bad news is that many of the refined foods that we commonly eat are the cause of insulin resistance. The good news is that you can prevent health problems by changing your eating habits. During recent years, scientific research has helped us to understand much more clearly which are the good foods and which are the bad foods. Insulin resistance is a disease of the cell receptors that have become worn out by too much sugar stimulation, which is why understanding some basic principles of "good eating" is crucial to maintaining and stabilizing the level of insulin in the blood.

Here are my nine principles for fighting insulin resistance:

1. Avoid refined carbohydrates, white flour, white rice, white sugar, and sweeteners.

2. Eat fresh, natural foods.

3. Remember that starchy vegetables such as potatoes and turnips are also a source of carbohydrates.

4. Keep your consumption of carbohydrates at a moderate or low level, according to your metabolic capacities. If you put on weight, cut down on sugar and carbohydrates, especially in the evening.

5. Avoid soft drinks, fruit juices (unless freshly squeezed), and alcohol.

6. Replace vegetable oils rich in omega-6 fatty acids and use virgin olive oil (guaranteed first cold pressing) instead.

7. Enrich your diet with omega-3 fatty acids by regularly eating oily fish, such as pink trout.

8. Be careful when it comes to foods with saturated fatty acids, found in fried foods, margarine, sweets, and cakes.

CHOOSE FOODS ACCORDING TO THE GLYCEMIC INDEX

The glycemic index is a measure based on the level of glucose entering the bloodstream once a carbohydrate has been absorbed. Diets rich in foods with a high glycemic index lead to insulin resistance. In contrast, diets consisting of foods with a low glycemic index prevent this phenomenon.

FOODS WITH A HIGH GLYCEMIC INDEX

- Most grains and their derivatives, such as white breads
- Breakfast cereals, muesli, porridge, and cereal bars
- Honey and sugar
- Most cookies, sweets, and snack bars
- Corn and potatoes, cooked carrots, and pumpkin
- Bananas and dried fruit

FOODS WITH A LOW TO MODERATE GLYCEMIC INDEX

- White beans, lentils, peas, chickpeas, and lima beans
- Dairy products such as milk and yogurt. However, be careful of the milk sugar galactose, which is an insulin stimulator. For those who want to lose weight, I suggest reducing the intake of dairy prod-

9. Eat protein or vegetable fat at each meal. Between meals, you can have a small amount of dark chocolate and avocado or pear.

Without a doubt, the most important part of my nutrition program lies in avoiding refined carbohydrates. Carbohydrates are directly linked to the development of insulin resistance and its consequences (diabetes and cardiovascular disease). You surely know that sugar quickly increases the level of glucose, but do you know that white flour, which is found in white bread as well as cookies and pastries, has exactly the same effect? White bread has a higher glycemic index (which measures the way the glucose level increases in the body) than sugar! In other words, white bread increases the glucose level further

---

ucts, except for all forms of cheese, which are essential for break-fast. For those whose aim is to prevent aging and who really like milk and natural yogurt, these can be eaten as a mid-afternoon snack, along with some fruit.

- Certain fruits, such as peaches, grapes, cherries, plums, grapefruit, kiwis, and mangoes
- Certain vegetables, such as beetroot and raw carrots

MORE FOODS WITH A LOW GLYCEMIC INDEX: NON-STARCHY VEGETABLES

These vegetables are dense at the nutritional level, providing lots of vitamins and minerals. They are digested slowly and have a low glycemic index on account of their high fiber content.

- Asparagus
- Bok choy
- Broccoli
- Cauliflower
- Celery
- Cucumber
- Green and yellow beans
- Green, red, and Chinese cabbage
- Lettuce, all types
- Mushrooms
- Spinach
- Sweet and hot peppers
- Tomatoes
- Zucchini

---

and more quickly than sugar. Any product containing white flour or white sugar has insufficient fiber to help the body effectively metabolize these carbohydrates. The same problem exists with white rice. There is also lots of hidden sugar in the sweeteners found in all sorts of refined foods, even so-called low-fat foods. The composition of foods is clearly labeled on food packages, so it is up to you to pay attention. Look particularly at the level of total carbohydrates on the nutrition label and try to choose foods with a relatively low level.

What I am proposing to you is the very same diet that protected our Paleolithic ancestors against insulin resistance: natural food, which comes directly from the vine and the field. If you eat whole and natural carbohydrates, your glucose and insulin levels will drop. On the other hand, if you eat processed carbohydrates, your glucose level will increase along with your insulin. The more a carbohydrate is processed, the fewer natural carbohydrate fibers it contains. Take the following example:

- A whole apple reduces glucose and insulin levels more than apple-sauce.

- Applesauce reduces glucose and insulin levels more than apple juice.

- Apple juice reduces glucose and insulin levels more than concentrated apple juice.

A whole apple is best at preventing insulin resistance because it is richest in fiber to slow down the entry of glucose into the bloodstream. Concentrated apple juice is the least desirable because it enters the bloodstream quickly, immediately stimulating the secretion of undesirable insulin.

Unrefined carbohydrates have another great advantage: they are much denser at the nutritional level than processed carbohydrates. They supply larger quantities of vitamins and minerals in proportion to their calories. For example, brown rice is denser at the nutritional level than white rice; fresh cooked beans are denser at the nutritional level than canned beans; and fresh vegetables are denser at the nutritional level than frozen vegetables.

Give priority to dense carbohydrates—such as whole grains, starchy vegetables (apart from potatoes), legumes, and fruit—but eat them in small quantities. This dietetic principle is often one of the hardest to understand because it supposes that all natural foods are healthy. Vegetables have four to six times fewer carbohydrates than foods based on grains, starch, and legumes. You can, therefore, eat lots of non-starchy vegetables without developing excess insulin.

RECOMMENDED SOURCES OF PROTEIN

Foods of animal origin—chicken, turkey, fish, seafood, rabbit and game, eggs, and low-fat cheeses—are all rich in protein. The best sources of animal proteins are from game such as venison, rabbit, and partridge, because in addition to being rich in protein, they contain little fat and are rich in micronutrients.

Here are a few pointers to help you select high-quality protein:

- When shopping, choose uncooked, unprepared cuts of chicken and turkey and lean cuts of lamb and beef. Eat poultry without the skin.

- Deep-fried meat and lardy products, hot dogs, sausages, bologna, other processed meats, and meat-based conserves didn't exist in the Paleolithic age. They are too rich in saturated fats and must be avoided.

- Legumes also contain protein, but they are much richer in carbo-hydrates than in protein, so eat them with caution. The same goes for seeds and grains, which also contain protein, but have a higher level of fat than protein. The fat they contain is healthy—mostly monounsaturated fatty acids—so a small helping of seeds or grains make relatively healthy snacks. Grains are slightly better than seeds because they generally tend to have a higher propor-tion of protein.

- Our Paleolithic ancestors never ate cheese and most cheese has a high fat level, much higher than its protein level. However, cheeses that are naturally low in fat, like mozzarella, feta, and low-fat *fro-mage blanc*, have good levels of protein.

FOODS TO AVOID THAT STIMULATE THE SECRETION OF INSULIN

These foods dramatically stimulate the pancreas to release insulin. They should, therefore, be completely avoided.

Alcoholic drinks (including aperitifs, strong alcohol, beer, and liqueurs)

Bacon

Bananas

Butter

Cakes

Cookies

Cereals (except whole-grain varieties)

Chocolate (except dark chocolate; containing at least 70 percent cocoa)

Coffee

Cream

Croissants (except at 4 P.M. for those who don't have weight to lose)

Dried fruits

Fast food

Foods with excessive animal fats

Fried food

Granola

Hard cheese (except feta, parmesan, and Romano)

Hot dogs

Ice cream

Jams and jellies

Mangoes

Margarine

Molasses

Muffins

Pancakes

Pastries

Peas

Pickles

Pizzas

Popcorn

Pudding

Pumpkin

Soft drinks (including commercial fruit juice)

Sorbet

Sponge cake

Sugar and sugary foods

Tacos

Tarts

Waffles

In terms of beverages, our Paleolithic ancestors drank little or no alcohol. They didn't have drinks that were rich in glucose, nor did they have fruit juice or caffeine-based drinks. They drank the only drink that is a food in itself: water. The most important thing is to avoid soft drinks. These drinks, which have only been available since the last century, are liquid sugar. And fruity drinks and fruit juices, although they appear to be healthy, contain the sugar of fruit without any of their regulating fiber. These two forms of drink attack the body's control of glucose and insulin regulation.

Research into alcohol has produced a hodgepodge of results: studies have shown that wine is good for health, but alcohol in general is metabolized by the body like carbohydrates. To understand the effects of alcohol on the body, just think of someone with a "beer belly." A beer belly is a clear sign of insulin resistance provoked by too many carbohydrates, which rapidly increase the levels of glucose and insulin. Alcohol, in other words, acts like sugar in the body. It damages brain and liver cells and can lead to a "fatty liver," which does not process fats correctly. It is, therefore, preferable to avoid alcohol, but you knew that already!

The healthiest drinks for our body are water and tea. You should try to use filtered or bottled water to avoid contaminants. Sparkling water, herbal teas, black tea, and green tea are also essential and beneficial choices. But be careful of black coffee, which increases the secretion of insulin and the level of the stress hormone cortisol. So, you now know where the surge of energy is coming from after your 11 A.M. coffee break!

Our Paleolithic ancestors' diet consisted of, on average, 30 percent protein; in the United States today, the average is only about 12 percent. Protein plays many critical roles in the body, including the stimulation of glucagons, a hormone that opposes insulin and allows the body to burn up stocks of carbohydrates, thereby creating energy. In other words, glucagon helps ameliorate the excessive production of insulin, stimulates the combustion of fats in the body, and maintains the equilibrium of glucose in the blood, so that the brain, heart, and kidneys function correctly (these organs cannot work properly without sugar).

If you want to prevent or reverse insulin resistance and lose weight, it is absolutely essential that you consume proteins in the correct proportion throughout the day. Unfortunately, many people don't think about food until they are very hungry, and then grab something quickly (which nearly always contains processed carbohydrates). To change your habits, you must think of proteins in dietetic terms: protein must be a key part of your diet. At home, be sure to eat a little high-quality protein throughout the day, preferably at each meal and sometimes in between.

All this brings an acceptable balance of sugar into the blood and prevents insulin resistance, avoiding the characteristic and often inexplicable problems of weight gain and fatigue that accompany this biological phenomenon.

It always comes back to what we eat!

Exactly. "We are what we eat"—this old saying is more topical than ever. Diet is the cornerstone of our health. All our hopes and risks depend upon it: we must learn to "eat better," which is, I repeat, not eating less but eating more at the right time.

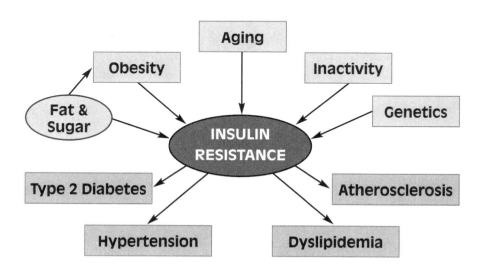

CHAPTER 5

The Problem of Food Allergies

JULIEN: *What is a food allergy?*

DR. CHAUCHARD: Food allergy is a problem with intestinal absorption of a particular food that leads to an inflammatory syndrome (again). It involves an excessive response of our immune system to the allergens of a particular food, which can provoke an allergic response (or hypersensitivity). Some foods are known to cause problems, such as dairy products, cereals, certain fish and seafood, certain fruits, and peanuts. Many airlines have even stopped serving peanuts, following too many allergic reactions from their passengers during the flight.

What are the symptoms?

We all know someone who suffers from allergy symptoms, such as noisy breathing, runny nose, irritable intestine, headache, or itching. Nearly 25 percent of the population has significant allergies to certain types of food, chemical products, or inhalants. The real incidence of these allergies is considerably higher if we include less serious symptoms such as occasional anxiety, generalized fatigue, dehydration, and other common afflictions. This phenomenon is widespread and yet little understood by the general public.

The symptoms can be so diverse and manifold that they become confusing. Symptoms can vary wildly from one individual to another in reaction to the same food, because everyone's immune response is different. What follows is a list of symptoms compiled to help you understand that some of your warning signs can be the result of an intolerant reaction to certain foods. However, it is important to remember that these symptoms can also be associated with other pathologies, and only your clinical history, medical examination, and laboratory tests can make the distinction.

What are the causes of allergies?

An unbalanced diet, stress, certain genetic predispositions, infections and inflammation, medicine, environmental pollution, chemical products, and toxins are all factors that can contribute to the development of food allergies or intolerances.

How will I know if I have allergies?

You will be delighted to know that most food allergies can be tested through a small blood sample. It is a quick and painless test carried out in a laboratory. You will easily discover what you must avoid or include in your diet and environment to reduce these allergies or intolerances as much as possible and give your body the time to rest and be cured. Allergic reactions lead to inflammatory reactions, especially in the intestine, and this inflammation in turn attacks the cell membranes.

When should I start to worry? What should I do about it?

You should immediately consult your doctor if you have bad itching, skin eruptions, or swellings shortly after a meal. You should write down everything you have consumed during the hours preceding the allergic incident, both medicine and food. Finally, if possible, you should freeze a small portion of the foods you have eaten.

Once a person has been diagnosed, in the case of itching or swollen lips, he or she must immediately take cortisol and antihistamines. If there are respiratory symptoms, a bronchodilator spray should be used. Finally, in the event of dizziness (losing consciousness or fainting), an adrenaline injection should be given immediately and an ambulance called for. There are only a few minutes in which to react! In other words, extreme reactions are serious, immediate, and triggered by proteins of immunoglobulin E (IgE), an antibody subclass.

SYMPTOMS ASSOCIATED WITH FOOD ALLERGY

DIGESTIVE SYSTEM

- Indigestion
- Nausea and vomiting
- Irritable intestine
- Diarrhea
- Constipation
- Flatulence
- Stomach ulcers
- Hemorrhoids
- Abdominal pain
- Colic (in babies)

URINARY TRACT

- Frequent need to urinate
- Burning sensation on urinating
- Urinary forgetfulness in children

CARDIOPULMONARY

- Asthma
- Irregular pulse

MUSCLES AND JOINTS

- Muscular pain
- Painful joints
- Joint inflammation (arthritis)
- Rheumatoid polyarthritis

COGNITIVE AND PSYCHOLOGICAL

- Mood swings
- Anxiety
- Depression
- Bulimia
- Loss of concentration
- Fatigue
- Hyperactivity
- Eccentric behavior in children

HEAD AND NECK

- Ear infections
- Runny nose or blocked nose
- Recurrent sinusitis
- Headaches/migraines
- Painful throat
- Mouth infections

OTHER SYMPTOMS

- Dehydration
- Weight gain
- Eczema
- Pins and needles sensation
- Skin eruptions
- Excessive sweating

As you can clearly see, many symptoms can be linked to food allergy. Furthermore, this list is not exhaustive. If your symptoms do not appear here, that doesn't mean that they are not due to food allergy. Now you will be wondering if your symptoms are allergic in origin . . .

Immunoglobulin G (IgG) reactions, on the other hand, have a twenty-four to forty-eight-hour delay, are less dangerous than IgE reactions, but are very tough on the digestive system. These delayed reactions grow weaker after stopping the allergen, and six months later it is common to no longer find IgG in the blood. On the contrary, IgE-type reactions are definitive in some individuals, they do not grow weaker, and continue to present the same risk, which may be life threatening.

How can we prevent allergic reactions to foods? What diet should we follow?

As soon as the foods you are allergic to have been identified, your doctor will help you with a program of elimination and reintroduction (the challenge phase). This program will determine which foods, if any, your body will reaccept. In the elimination phase, you remove from your diet the foods to which you react. The challenge phase begins after the elimination and consists of reintroducing these foods gradually into your diet.

The selection of foods for the challenge phase, or reintroduction, must be carried out methodically and in minute detail. These foods need to be reintroduced one by one and any symptoms duly noted. First of all, you must reintegrate foods with a high nutritional value and those least likely to provoke a reaction. As soon as you have introduced these foods and observed your symptoms, you can then test other foods. This is important because every time an allergic phenomenon reappears, you lose the time it takes for your system to return to normal. Moreover, each "challenging" food must be reintroduced in its simplest form. For example, if you're trying to test your reaction to cow's milk, drink a glass of cow's milk, don't have a glass of hot chocolate. If you are testing corn, eat corn on the cob without butter, salt, or pepper and don't consume it with other foods.

Symptoms emerge at varying time scales—sometimes it takes up to three days for reactions to appear—according to the type of food, so it is recommended to wait a while between testing different foods. No food must be reintroduced at a time when a reaction to another food is possible, otherwise the reaction will be concealed. Wait for any reaction to die down before reintroducing a new food. If the symptoms appear after having absorbed certain foods, don't continue to eat these foods during the rest of the "challenge" period. Once again, that will disguise your results! The process of reintroduction is interesting, but delicate. You will learn more about food, your body, and your health, and going forward, you will have the results in hand.

Once you have identified the foods that are causing a reaction, thanks to the process of testing, elimination, and challenge, the next stage for you and your doctor is to choose a method of treatment. A specific treatment could include a change of diet, food supplements, or even a series of injections, if required. After treatment, you will no doubt again be capable of eating those foods you used to react to.

Is food allergy always apparent from the first contact with the food in question?

You can eat a food for years without it provoking a reaction in you. An allergy can suddenly develop at any moment to a food that your body used to tolerate perfectly well. On the other hand, some people will discover they are allergic to a particular food the first time they eat it.

Are the allergic symptoms always apparent immediately after eating the food in question?

The symptoms of allergy (skin, respiratory, or digestive) can develop within seconds, hours, or even days after eating the food. There are no rules and each person reacts differently.

Is it possible to become desensitized in order to get over a food allergy?

At present, no desensitization exists for food allergy. Therefore, the treatment of excluding the allergen is purely nutritional—it involves total elimination of the food responsible for the allergy.

Which foods are most likely to cause an allergic reaction?

Milk, peanuts, eggs, fish, shellfish, meat and lunch meats, vegetables, spices, certain fresh and dried fruits, soy, wheat, strawberries, apples, peaches, avocados, kiwis, bananas, chestnuts, celery, carrots, walnuts, hazelnuts, sesame seeds, sunflower seeds, yeast, figs, potatoes, lentils, peas, pork, chicken, rice . . . The list of foods likely to cause allergy is interminable!

One patient, Anne-Christine, age forty-eight, had been suffering for ten years from a chronic cough, which hadn't improved in spite of endless consultations. Her brother recommended my clinic. The results showed she had strong allergies to dairy products, prawns, corn, oats, sesame, and rice. Among the fruits she reacted strongly to were bananas, grapes, and pears. She also had a modest reaction to egg whites. By following a rotation diet adapted to her specific needs, her health improved spectacularly. And after just one visit, she no longer felt the need to return because her cough had completely disappeared.

Are children allergic to cow's milk?

There are five large groups of foods that represent three-quarters of food allergies in children: eggs, peanuts, milk, fish and shellfish, and various nuts. But children, like adults, can also be intolerant to many other foods.

Should we diversify an infant's diet at an early stage in order to avoid food allergy or intolerance later on?

This fashion from the 1970s and 1980s is responsible for much of the food allergy and intolerance in children today. The introduction of foods other than mother's milk before the age of four months increases by 150 percent the risk of getting eczema at the age of two. Today, pediatricians and allergy specialists advise delaying this diversification of infant food, and introducing the foods one by one, slowly and pro-gressively, especially in children whose parents have allergies.

What are the so-called cross-allergies?

Cross-allergies or cross-reactions are surprising but are being identified more and more. They develop between substances that do not appear to have any connection, like pollens, latex, and certain foods. For exam-ple, you must be careful of kiwis if you are allergic to latex; this is a clas-sic cross-allergic reaction. If you are intolerant of latex, which is what surgical gloves and condoms are made of, you risk having reactions to one of the following foods: bananas, kiwis, avocados, chestnuts, figs, passion fruit, cherries, apricots, or papayas. Someone allergic to dust mites may develop a food allergy to snails. If you are allergic to birch pollen, be careful of apples, hazelnuts, walnuts and almonds, peaches, apricots, nectarines, celery, carrots, potatoes, and kiwis. Finally, an allergy to bird feathers can provoke a food allergy to eggs.

Is it true that globalization may be a source of certain forms of food allergy?

The development of a food allergy depends on a combination of factors, both genetic and environmental. And this last century has seen a real revolution in our eating habits, which is partly responsible for an explosive increase in intolerance. Due to globalization, we have access to fast foods, exotic products and spices, and restaurants that serve every form of international food—our diet has considerably evolved and has opened up to "world food," for better or for worse. One negative consequence has been a too early diversification of the infant diet.

TAKE ACTION AGAINST FOOD ALLERGIES

- If you are aware that you have an extreme reaction to a particular food, don't try to "challenge" it without the supervision of a medical specialist.

- The key to a long-term cure is finding the underlying causes of your allergy or intolerance.

- Speak to your doctor, because he or she will carry out the widest range of blood tests for food allergy (more than ninety-six foods, twenty-four herbs, and twenty-four spices are covered), so that none can go uncovered. These tests are quick and effective, and they have helped me solve so many cases that I can only be enthusiastic about them.

Getting rid of food allergy is a big step forward, not only for good digestion, but also for beautiful skin and a more energetic life.

The changes in techniques used by the food industry, including pasteurization, freezing, and the addition of flavorings and colorings, means that what we eat today is a far cry from the traditional chicken casserole of yesteryear. If for the majority of us this change in habits comes with many advantages such as increased food choices, for those who have inherited a genetic disposition to allergy, it can soon become a nightmare. And the number of people with food allergies is growing.

Does genetic modification of crops risk intensifying food allergy?

It's too early to say. In practice, we haven't noticed any specific allergy to genetically modified (GM) food. In fact, the genetic modification of certain food proteins could even be seen as a good thing. For example, in peanuts, if we managed to modify the protein that causes allergy, we could imagine one day eating this food without risk.

Is there any prospect of a code of conduct for the food industry?

Allergy specialists are fighting to obtain clear labeling of products, at least as far as nuts are concerned. Generally, we're seeing more allergy warnings on food labels, so the information is getting out there.

CHAPTER 6

Free Radicals and the "Rusting" Body

JULIEN: *If I understand correctly, the "serial killers" of our cell membranes and our genetic code are the cytokines, generated by the inflammatory mechanism. Is our organism under threat from any other public enemy number one?*

DR. CHAUCHARD: Of course—the free radicals. Above all, as we get older, free radicals are increasingly active in destroying our cells. This phenomenon is known as oxidation, which also leads to inflammation.

Don't tell me I'm getting rusty! How do you explain the phenomenon of oxidation in our body?

Human aging is largely modulated by the processes using energy. In fact, when we produce energy, we are burning up the fuels (made up of sugar and animal fats) in the fire of the oxygen that we breathe. This combustion is imperfect. It allows unstable molecules—free radicals—to escape from the mitochondria. (Mitochondria are present in large numbers in the cells' cytoplasm and are where energy is produced.) These free radicals attack the other constituent parts of living matter and cause a real molecular "rusting," which spares none of the elements that make up our cells.

Oxidation is actually a perfectly natural phenomenon of the cell because oxidizing oxygen is what we do to produce energy. Oxidation happens when oxygen is added to a substance and, thereby, stimulates a chemical change and release of energy. In this sense, we can say that it is the very carburetor that is making us live that, in some way, also destroys us, by "rusting" us. Our cell membranes oxidize and the fatty acids of these membranes go "rancid"—that is, they lose their elasticity.

How do the free radicals operate?

For the most part, free radicals are oxygen molecules that have lost an electron, thereby gaining energy. These free radicals flee to the DNA molecules and the cell walls to acquire their stability. Because a free-radical molecule is missing an electron, it creates a negative charge. Because of this energy imbalance, the free radical attaches itself to another, balanced molecule to try to steal an electron from it. In this way, the balanced molecule becomes, in turn, unbalanced and so becomes a free radical itself, and further reactions quickly follow. This chain reaction causes damage all along the way.

What are the ill effects we can expect free radicals to have on the organism?

Oxidation affects all our tissues, all the cell groups that make up the human body: muscles, skin, liver, kidneys, stomach, intestine, brain, genitals, and so on. Free radicals attack the structure of the cell membranes, thus creating metabolic waste. Their toxic accumulation interferes with the communication of cells, disrupts the DNA, the RNA, and the synthesis of proteins, lowers energy levels, and, in general, gets in the way of vital chemical processes. In other words, free radicals negatively affect the entire functioning of the cell.

They damage healthy cells and are responsible for many degenerative diseases, such as atherosclerosis, cataracts, degeneration of the retina, Alzheimer's disease, and cancer. They are at the root of the aging process: wearing out the joints (cartilage, ligaments, tendons); drying the skin (wrinkles, age spots); weakening the muscular tissues; and increasing symptoms linked to age (lessening of the cognitive faculties, loss of strength). These dangerous oxidant molecules also play a very important role in the aging of the skin.

The disasters caused by free radicals evolve surreptitiously over the years, without showing any sign of their destructive work. When the disease appears, it is already late (but not too late) to intervene. It is then necessary to strengthen the body with effective antioxidants to combat the aggressors.

What forms of behavior encourage the production of free radicals?

Free radicals are produced naturally in the body, as a result of energy production in the mitochondria: the simple acts of living, eating, and breathing create them. Other free radicals come from external causes—combustion fumes, chemical products, ionizing radiation, electromagnetic rays, pesticides, solvents, tobacco, alcohol, sun rays, pollution, asbestos, chlorine, ozone, and certain drugs. Finally, an overly rich diet and a badly managed lifestyle accelerate the production of free radicals within the body.

How can we protect ourselves from free radicals?

You see now that free radicals are formed, upon contact with oxygen, by the body itself, and we can't do anything to stop that. To counteract the disastrous consequences of these substances, our body naturally produces antioxidant enzymes, such as superoxide dismutase (SOD), myeloperoxidase, and catalase. The free radicals produced are less dangerous if the body makes enough antioxidants and our diet supports our anti-free-radical defenses.

A young body in good condition is capable of fighting off the invasion of free radicals by making its own antioxidants. But the older we get, the less capable our body is of defending itself against them. It is necessary to consume a maximum of foods that are rich in antioxidants or even, in certain cases, to take food supplements that contain antioxidants.

To break up the free radicals, the body also calls on nutrients like vitamins C and E, the amino acids taurine and cysteine, and the minerals zinc and selenium. These substances attach themselves to the free radicals and neutralize them, thereby diminishing the attacks on our cells.

What is the role of antioxidants?

By intercepting the oxidant agents, the antioxidants inhibit the chain reaction responsible for the formation of new free radicals. But their action doesn't stop there—they can also repair damage. Antioxidants stop the damage caused by destructive agents that haven't been eradicated in time and they eliminate and replace the molecules that have been damaged. After their fight against free radicals, they clean up the battlefield and destroy the undesirable substances created by their activities.

Antioxidants belong to one of three categories:

- *Preventive agents*—Their role is to annihilate the molecules of endogenous (inside the organism) or exogenous (outside the organism) origin that are responsible for producing free radicals.

- *Agents of active detoxification*—There are three specific enzymes produced by the body: superoxide dismutase, or SOD (which inhibits chain reactions), catalase (which oxidizes toxins), and myeloperoxidase (which takes charge of the detoxification of carcinogenic agents).

- *Agents of passive detoxification*—Exogenic in origin, they eliminate a part of the free radicals that have resisted the first two defenses (prevention agents and active detoxification agents). The best-known are beta-carotene (a precursor to vitamin A) and vitamins C and E. They can be found in most fruits and vegetables (beta-carotene and C) or vegetable oils (vitamin E). There are also the antioxidants zinc, selenium, and lycopene (from tomatoes) that we obtain from our food.

The benefit of increasing our consumption of antioxidants has been proven, and these nutrients actively participate to prevent the diseases that accompany our advancing years.

When should we add supplements to our diet?

When we are young, the fact that we consume on a daily basis foods containing antioxidants gives our body the necessary weapons to combat free radicals. When we get older, this is no longer sufficient, and we need a large dose of external antioxidants to limit the damage.

Recent work carried out all over the world shows that antioxidants can prevent many of the "corrosion" phenomena provoked by free radicals and the unstable derivatives of oxygen. We are now seeing the arrival in health food stores of GliSODin (superoxide dismutase), the first product of its kind that can be taken by mouth and which seems to be excellent for slowing down cellular damage.

If you want to be able to undertake your favorite physical activity throughout your life while allowing your body to repair, when necessary, the damage that vigorous exercise can cause, you must take a good antioxidant supplement containing the following nutrients:

- Beta-carotene or vitamin A (for destruction of cancerous agents)

- Selenium (for neutralizing free radicals)

- Vitamin E, if possible in the form of tocotrienols (for using oxygen and protecting tissues against oxidation)

- Vitamin C, a minimum of 1 gram per day (for elimination of free radicals and stimulation of the immune system)

Be careful to avoid synthetic food supplements. Some of them are mutagenic or even carcinogenic. Instead, choose natural food supplements.

What proof do we have that antioxidant supplements are beneficial?

Every week, new results are published that confirm the importance of adequate doses of antioxidants. Here's a sampling:

- Taking supplements of vitamins A, C, and E plus zinc is associated with a reduced risk of prostate cancer in an epidemiological study carried out on 1,363 people.

- Elderly people in an institution who took a supplement of selenium and zinc for two years had significantly fewer respiratory infections, according to a French study.

- People over age sixty-five who take a daily vitamin and mineral supplement see an improvement in their immediate memory, attention span, and ability to solve problems, according to a recent Canadian study.

- An Italian study shows that people aged 100 in good health have higher blood levels of the antioxidant vitamins C and E than a comparable population aged seventy to ninety-nine.

- In 442 people in good health, between sixty-five and ninety-four years old, it is the levels of vitamin C and beta-carotene that appear to be predictors of the best cognitive performance.

- Patients suffering from various forms of dementia or Alzheimer's disease have lower levels of antioxidant vitamins than people in good health.

- When 633 people over age sixty-five in good health were assessed and then reassessed, on average, fifty-two months later, 91 of them presented signs of dementia. Among regular consumers of vitamins C or E, no case of dementia was registered.

- In a study carried out on over 88,000 women, the regular taking of multivitamin supplements diminishes by 26 percent the risk of breast cancer among those who consume more than 15 grams of alcohol per day.

By simply taking antioxidant supplements, it is possible to fight off early death. We might even hope to spectacularly increase our average life expectancy or even the maximum life expectancy of our species (at present, 120 years). At least we'll all be a little less "rusty" . . .

What is the role of vitamin E, and how much should we take?

Taking vitamin E diminishes the risk of coronary illness by reducing the aggregation of blood platelets. A controlled study of vitamin E, carried out on 2,000 patients with coronary illness, showed that this vitamin reduced the risk of heart attack by 75 percent. Taking 400 IU per day of vitamin E will reduce by 30 to 40 percent the risk of coronary illness. The risk of having a stroke is reduced by half in those who take a vitamin supplement containing vitamin E, compared to those who do not take it, according to another study. The list of advantages of vitamin E supplementation go on:

- According to studies, the benefits of vitamin E could also extend to the prevention of prostate cancer, jaw decay, Parkinson's disease, and Alzheimer's disease.

- The administration of 2,000 IU of vitamin E a day in moderate cases of Alzheimer's disease delays by 230 days (compared with a placebo) the loss of autonomy, institutionalization, or death.

- The immune functions of older people are clinically improved by supplements of vitamin E, and it is recommended that the dose of this vitamin be increased with age.

- Smokers and ex-smokers over forty who take vitamin E (100 IU per day, at minimum) have a risk of prostate cancer (metastatic or fatal) that is 56 percent less than whose who do not take it.

Tocotrienol is one form of vitamin E that comes from whole rice, barley, and palm oil. Its particular benefit is that it penetrates the blood-brain barrier and protects brain cells.

A balanced diet should be sufficient for fulfilling your needs for vitamin E, estimated at 10–15 IU per day. If you smoke, you can safely take more, a supplement of 400–600 IU per day. I typically recommend 800 IU of the tocotrienol form of vitamin E per day.

What does selenium do?

Selenium is a trace element that activates the enzyme systems capable of neutralizing free radicals and it plays a part in metabolism as well. Because soil is becoming poorer with the use of chemical fertilizers, selenium is now in short supply in our diets.

A lot of recent studies underline the links between selenium deficiency and certain pathologies connected with aging. The healthy functioning of the brain appears to depend on a sufficient supply of selenium, which is indispensable to combat the oxidative stress of the

FOODS RICH IN ANTIOXIDANTS
AND OTHER IMPORTANT NUTRIENTS

The principal antioxidants are the minerals zinc, selenium, and copper, and the vitamins A, E, C, and B complex. The following list of foods will help you incorporate more antioxidants and other important nutrients into your diet:

- *Foods rich in calcium, without too much phosphorus:* yogurt, sardines and herring on the bone, salmon, tofu, almonds, cabbage, and broccoli

- *Foods rich in magnesium:* nuts, green vegetables, whole-grain cereals, oily fish, and certain shellfish like snails

- *Foods rich in potassium:* bananas, legumes, avocados, asparagus, carrots, lettuce, and whole-grain cereals

- *Foods rich in zinc:* oysters, poultry, fish, shellfish, chicken liver, eggs, and ginger

- *Foods rich in iron:* certain types of mineral water, chicken liver, oysters, dried fruit, spinach, and legumes

- *Foods rich in selenium:* Brazil nuts, seafood, chicken liver, whole-grain cereals, red peppers, wild mushrooms, and garlic

- *Foods rich in iodine:* shellfish, fish, and seaweed

- *Foods rich in silicium:* whole-grain cereals and some mineral waters

- *Foods rich in ascorbic acid (vitamin C):* spinach, peppers, watercress, parsley, chives, guava, papaya, kiwi, black currants, red currants, strawberries, oranges, lemons, grapefruit, and grapes

- *Foods rich in beta-carotene (pro-vitamin A):* cooked carrots, pumpkin, spinach, lettuce, watercress, melon, watermelon, mango, apricot, and prunes

- *Foods rich in lycopene:* tomato sauce, cooked tomatoes, watermelon, papaya, and pink grapefruit

- *Foods rich in lutein and zeaxanthin:* corn, broccoli, and green vegetables

- *Foods rich in tocopherols (vitamin E):* almonds, hazelnuts, and wheat germ

- *Foods rich in flavonoids:* onions, apples, blueberries, grapes, and blackberries

- *Vegetables rich in sulfur:* broccoli, Brussels sprouts, cauliflower, white cabbage, red cabbage, and Chinese cabbage

- *Foods rich in thiamine (vitamin B_1):* whole-grain cereal and legumes

- *Foods rich in folic acid (vitamin B_9):* spinach, watercress, lettuce, and asparagus

- Eat liver and fish rich in vitamins, especially in thiamine (B_1), niacin (B_3), pyridoxine (B_6), folic acid (B_9), and cobalamin (B_{12}).

- Eat fresh fruits and vegetables in every form: raw, juiced, pureed, and in soups, gazpacho, sauces, and lightly cooked compotes.

neurotransmitters. According to a French study, an accelerated decline of cognitive functions is observed in old people whose blood plasma is low in selenium. One study carried out on 1,312 subjects showed that a daily supplement of 200 micrograms (mcg) of selenium reduced the risk of prostate cancer by 63 percent, colon cancer by 58 percent, and lung cancer by 46 percent.

Selenium is found in foods that are rich in protein and sulfur—fish, cereals, and certain meats. Taking selenium as a supplement is not dangerous, provided you don't exceed 500 mcg per day. The recommended daily dose for an adult with no risk factors is 75–200 mcg. I would suggest a minimum of 200 mcg per day.

What is the effect of vitamin C?

Vitamin C's effect is widespread: it invigorates the immune system and stimulates psychomotor activity, and it also acts as a trap for free radicals. Consuming 300–400 milligrams (mg) of vitamin C (ascorbic acid) every day increases life expectancy by about six years in men and one year in women. Certain studies also show that men who consume a lot of vitamin C have overall mortality (death from all causes) that is 42 percent lower than those who consume little vitamin C, while their cardiac mortality is 45 percent lower.

Many studies point out the preventive action of ascorbic acid supplementation on cardiovascular pathologies. By taking vitamin C for a long period, we can significantly reduce high triglycerides, which can alone cause cardiovascular disease. For those in good health, taking supplements of vitamin C (2 grams per day) reduces the rigidity of the arteries and aggregation of the platelets, two conditions associated with a risk of atherosclerosis.

Excess of lead, a neurotoxin, is very damaging to overall health. Compared to smokers who don't take supplements, those who take vitamin C (1 gram per day) see the lead levels in their blood fall by 81 percent. Aging brings an increased risk of cataracts, and vitamin C can halve or even reduce by three-quarters the risk of developing this eye disease.

The recommended dose for an adult with no risk factors is 500 milligrams to 1 gram of vitamin C per day.

What is the role of beta-carotene and vitamin A?

Taken alongside vitamin E or selenium, vitamin A, or its precursor beta-carotene, protects cell membranes against free radicals. According to certain studies, it can also prevent cancers of the esophagus and the stomach. Men over forty years old who eat little fruit and vegetables but take a beta-carotene supplement (20 mg per day) have a 32 percent lower risk of prostate cancer than those who don't.

The daily quantities of vitamin A for an adult with no risk factors is 5 mg for women and 10–15 mg for men.

Are antioxidants a miracle cure?

Antioxidant supplements are just one of the elements at our disposal in reducing our risk of developing disease as we grow older. We have sufficient proof of their benefits to encourage all adults to increase their intake of vitamins C and E, zinc, and selenium. All these nutrients participate in the prevention of chronic diseases that increase with age and are probably linked to oxidant damage.

Healthy eating is always critical. In light of studies showing that overeating accelerates aging while restricting calorie intake slows it down, many of us in the healthcare profession have been advising patients for several years to choose foods that are nutritionally rich and to limit intake of empty calories, which increase oxidative stress. In particular, it is important to limit consumption of refined foods between meals; these include soft drinks, chocolate bars, and pastries. Here are some basic guidelines for healthy eating:

- Eat more foods containing antioxidant vitamins, minerals, and other nutrients (see "Foods Rich in Antioxidants and Other Important Nutrients" on page 68).

- I recommend regular consumption of spinach, broccoli, or cabbage, which are rich in beta-carotene.

- Take supplements combining selenium with other antioxidants such as vitamins E, A, and C, as well as zinc. Make sure these products are made by a reputable company to ensure potency. Look on the Internet site www.antiage-solutions.com for the best antioxidants and nutritional and anti-inflammatory products.

"FREE RADICAL" DISEASES

Diseases Associated with Free-Radical Damage

- Alzheimer's disease
- Atherosclerosis
- Cancer
- Cataracts
- Diabetes mellitus
- Essential hypertension
- Fanconi's anemia
- Parkinson's disease

CHAPTER 7

Glycation and Accelerated Aging

JULIEN: *Inflammation, oxidation, and . . . Things always come in threes. What other phenomenon are you going to reveal? We become inflamed, we get rusty . . .*

DR. CHAUCHARD: . . . and we caramelize. Glycation, or non-enzymatic glycosylation, is the third (after inflammation and oxidation) and least understood of the fundamental mechanisms of aging. We are threatened not only by interior rusting and decaying cell membranes but also by the insidious caramelization of our proteins due to chronically high levels of glucose in the blood. Glycation is a phenomenon that is just as threatening as the problems caused by oxygen and free radicals.

Caramelizing? It sounds like a culinary phenomenon . . .

Exactly. The speed of reaction depends upon the temperature. When cooking foods at high temperature (over 100°C/210°F, but especially over 180°C/355°F) in the oven or in a pan, something called Strecker's degradation occurs, making the food brown and giving it that smell particular to grilled food. Foods cooked this way are pro-inflammatory and may be carcinogenic. In this way, eating a well-grilled steak is the equivalent in terms of toxicity to smoking ten cigarettes! It is, therefore, not surprising that cancers of the digestive system have been linked to frequent consumption of grilled meat. Grilled vegetables are less toxic but should still be avoided. First immediate conclusion: Avoid overcooked food at barbeques!

Briefly, how do you explain the phenomenon of glycation?

Where there is excess sugar in the blood, the glucose molecules react with proteins—this is the phenomenon known as glycation. Glycation is the accumulation of sugar and proteins around the joints, muscles, and the skin. These bonds rigidify the collagen, the intercellular protein of our connective tissue, which makes the tissues stiffer and discourages communication between cells. The glycation of the proteins of the vascular walls makes them lose some of their mechanical properties, and they become resistant to the enzymes necessary for remodelling the walls. So, it's not just hardening of the arteries but hardening of the whole body that occurs with this carmelization process.

What are the effects of glycation on the body?

Glycation threatens to make us stiff as a poker! Cross-linking of collagen causes, for example, the loss of elasticity in the skin. Healthy collagen is normally made up of layers that maintain the skin's elasticity. Glycation acts in this way on all parts of the body and can destroy other vital organs, including the kidneys, lungs, and brain. Glycation is, therefore, a factor in the accelerated aging of tissue.

The products issued by glycation—called advanced glycation end products (AGEs)—accumulate with age and participate in the development of several diseases, such as atherosclerosis, kidney insufficiency, Alzheimer's disease, and cataracts. AGEs are particularly numerous in diabetics. So, when the proteins from the crystalline lens of the eye are damaged, a cataract may develop, or when the collagen supporting the arteries is affected, the risk of atherosclerosis increases dramatically.

This protein-sugar combination also stimulates the expression of adhesion molecules and sets off pro-coagulant activity, or increased blood clotting. It also initiates the secretion of extracellular messengers (cytokines, growth factors, and so on), which can be the starting point for an inflammatory reaction as well as vascular and neuronal deterioration. We, therefore, find the three phenomena linked together: glycation, oxidation, and inflammation.

Eating and breathing means dying a little: the two molecules that we desperately need, glucose and oxygen, end up making us age more quickly.

Is there any way of fighting against this phenomenon of glycation?

At present, apart from controlling our glycemic balance over the long term and reducing as far as possible our consumption of burnt foods, the only substances allowing us to struggle against the harmful effects of AGEs are carnosine, aminoguanidine, and lipoic acid. Carnosine is a natural atoxic molecule that intervenes at the first stages of the glycation process to form inoffensive products that are quickly eliminated; aminoguanidine is a chemical inhibitor; and lipoic acid helps keep the levels of sugar in the blood under control and thereby diminish glycation.

What are the benefits of carnosine and how much should one take?

The age-preventative properties of carnosine, a natural protein found in the skeletal muscle and the brain, have recently been proven. Carnosine is an anti-glycation molecule that acts against lesions created by sugar. High levels of carnosine are present in the long-life cells (such as neurons), and the concentration of muscular carnosine is positively correlated to longevity.

There is a high level of carnosine in muscles that actively contract and a low level is found in certain cases of muscular disease, such as Duchenne's disease. Muscular carnosine concentration diminishes with age, showing the benefit of taking carnosine supplements as we grow older.

Most important is carnosine's anti-glycation effect. Carnosine reacts with sugars (glucose, galactose, dihydroxyacetone) to form glycic carnosine, a nontoxic substance that the body can then eliminate. In addition, carnosine inactivates the glycic proteins through its reaction with dihydroxyacetone. Carnosine helps to reduce the glycation of proteins and the formation of AGEs by improving the recognition of these products by their receptors.

In one study, a daily dose of 50 milligrams (mg) of carnosine taken by twenty healthy volunteers for one to four months showed several positive effects: half the subjects remarked upon the benefits to their facial appearance, their muscular resistance, or their general well-being, while some noticed an improvement in terms of sleeping and libido. These benefits appeared in a short time, whereas the expected effect for age-prevention would only be noticed after long-term use of the supplement.

Carnosine is also an antioxidant that protects and stabilizes the cell membrane, much like vitamin E. High levels of free radicals and toxins have been inactivated by taking carnosine supplements. It also stimulates the maturation of immunocompetent cells and reduces inflammation. Carnosine, therefore, fights against oxidation, glycation, and inflammation, whereas other substances only act against one of these factors. Carnosine would be effective not only in prevention but also in therapy.

For age-prevention, I typically recommend doses of 100–200 mg per day. But to treat certain diseases and, notably, when it is used to fight against the secondary effects of chemotherapy for cancer, daily doses of 3,000 mg of carnosine can be used.

What are the benefits of aminoguanidine?

Aminoguanidine improves the elasticity of the arteries. It combines with the early products of glycation to form a reactive composition. Aminoguanidine acts on the retina, the kidneys, and the neurons. In the retina, it prevents the formation of AGEs in the microvessels and the formation of micro-aneurysms, and it inhibits the development of diabetic retinopathy. In the kidneys, it prevents the formation of AGEs in the glomeruli (clusters of capillaries found at each nephron tubule in the kidney and held together by connective tissue), and reduces by 90 percent the excretion of the protein albumin in diabetics. In the neurons, it eliminates diabetic neuropathy by preventing a reduction of the conducting speed of the nervous influx, normalizing the amplitude of potential action and the sanguine flux reaching the peripheral nerves. For age prevention, I typically recommend doses of 250–500 mg of aminoguanidine per day.

What about the role of lipoic acid?

Lipoic acid plays an important role in cellular aging because it reduces the protein damage linked to excess sugar by facilitating the conversion of blood sugar (glucose) into energy. A derivative, dihydrolipoic acid, is called a universal antioxidant: it is very well absorbed by the digestive system and is then diffused through all the tissues, neutralizing free radicals and generating other antioxidants.

Lipoic acid also has the unique ability to protect the DNA from free radicals and also help repair oxidized DNA. Lipoic acid has been successfully used in Germany in the treatment of diabetes, for thirty-five years. Taking lipoic acid speeds up the transport of glucose by stimulating its transporters. In 1995, a conference on diabetic neuropathy concluded that lipoic acid was the agent of choice for the prevention of diabetic complications (neuropathy, cardiomyopathy, and retinopathy). For age prevention, I typically recommend doses of 100–300 mg lipoic acid per day.

CHAPTER 8

Good Fats Keep the Body Young

JULIEN: *Now that I know about all the phenomena and fundamental factors of aging, I'm keen to start on your 30-day health program . . .*

DR. CHAUCHARD: Good. A patient who is aware and willing is already halfway there. But before starting the program, I want to discuss fatty acids (FAs). You need to know that there are all sorts of fats, but I will talk to you mostly about omega-3 and omega-6 fatty acids. Their efficacy in our struggle against aging will depend on a good nutritional balance between these two.

What are the characteristics of these fatty acids?

Fatty acids are either saturated or unsaturated, according to whether their molecules are capable of attaching themselves to other molecules. Oils are each composed of a variable proportion of saturated and unsaturated FAs.

The more they are composed of saturated FAs, the more stable the oils are in the presence of light and heat. The extreme case is palm oil: its FAs are so naturally saturated (refinement also allows the artificial saturation of oils) that at room temperature it comes in a solid and not a liquid form. These so-called stable oils are used for cooking and frying.

In contrast, the richer they are in unsaturated FAs, the more fragile they are—under the effects of heat and light, they can turn rancid very quickly. This is the case with walnut oil, which can only be used cold in salads, away from the light.

The unsaturated FAs are divided between monounsaturated and polyunsaturated FAs. Olive oil is well balanced in these different fatty acids, which is why it is good for cooking or in salads. The famous Mediterranean diet recommends two tablespoons per day in a mix of olive oil (60 percent) and canola oil (40 percent). There are also monounsaturated FAs in foods such as avocados, foie gras, goose, and duck fat.

Polyunsaturated fatty acids (PUFAs) are classed in two groups: the omega-6s are present above all in sunflower oil, corn oil, and grapeseed oil; the omega-3s are present in walnuts, canola oil, purslane, and oily fish. These polyunsaturated fatty acids (omega-3s and omega-6s) partake in important processes like the constitution and integration of cell membranes, the functioning of the cardiovascular system and the brain, the composition of hormones, as well as the regulation of the inflammatory processes.

Certain fatty acids are said to be "essential" because the body cannot make them by itself. It, therefore, has to get them from foods or supplements.

Can you tell me more about omega-3s?

Many studies show that people are lacking in omega-3 FAs, as well as being short on antioxidants and magnesium. The omega-3s participate in maintaining the cell membranes, playing an essential role in intercellular communication (for example, in the memory functions of the brain), and promoting the suppleness of our blood vessels, skin, and joints. They play a central role at the cell membrane level and intervene in numerous biochemical processes in the body: the regulation of blood pressure, the immune and anti-inflammatory reactions, and the aggregation of blood platelets.

Of the omega-3s, only alpha-linolenic acid (ALA) is said to be "essential." The other omega-3 FAs can be produced by the body. ALA is particularly present in flaxseed and flaxseed oil, in hemp and its oil, and in canola oil.

Another member of the omega-3 family is eicosapentaenoic acid (EPA). Our body can synthesize it through ALA, but we can also get it directly from certain foods, notably oily fish. Populations that consume a lot of fish (the Inuits of Greenland and the Japanese, for example) are much less affected by cardiovascular disease, due to higher levels of EPA in their diets.

Finally, docosahexaenoic acid (DHA), another omega-3, is also present in seafood, particularly oily fish. DHA plays a fundamental role in the development of the brain and the retina as well as the formation and mobility of sperm.

What dose of omega-3 is necessary?

Omega-3s and their properties are the subject of hundreds of research projects each year, which contribute to the evolution of nutritional advice. A certain number of countries, as well as the World Health Organization, have provided recommendations for omega-3 intake. They are as follows:

- ALA: from 0.8 to 1.1 gram (g) per day
- EPA + DHA: from 0.3 to 0.5 g per day

There are a number of food sources of omega-3 fatty acids as well. To obtain the necessary daily omega-3s, include one of the following foods in your diet each day.

Omega-3s of vegetable origin (ALA)

- ½ teaspoon of flaxseed oil
- 2 teaspoons of crushed flaxseed
- 1 tablespoon of canola oil
- ½ cup of nuts
- 13 g of hemp seeds

Omega-3s of marine origin (EPA + DHA)

- 2.5 ounces of salmon (Alaskan or organically farmed)
- 3.15 ounces of pink or red salmon (canned)
- 3.15 ounces of sardines
- 4.2 ounces of white tuna

Other good marine sources of omega-3s include Atlantic halibut, fresh herring, trout, mackerel, unsalted fresh anchovies, red mullet, John Dory, and capelin, among others.

Can you tell me more about omega-6s?

Omega-6 FAs play an important role in the nervous system, in cardio-vascular balance, in immunity and healing wounds, and in allergic and inflammatory reactions. Consumed in excess, the omega-6 FAs can prevent the omega-3 FAs from playing their role, notably in cardiovas-cular protection, and provoke pains and inflammatory diseases like asthma or arthritis.

Of the omega-6s, only linoleic acid (LA) is said to be "essential." The other omega-6 fatty acids can be made by the body from LA. In contrast to ALA, linoleic acid is abundantly present in the modern diet: in corn oil, sunflower oil, soy oil, grapeseed oil, and so on.

Another member of the omega-6 family is gamma-linolenic acid (GLA). The body synthesizes GLA from linoleic acid, but several obsta-cles can harm this conversion: excess cholesterol, excess bad fats (trans-fats, saturated fats, and so on), alcohol, aging, and diabetes. We can get it directly from borage oil (24 percent GLA), evening primrose oil (9 percent GLA), black currant oil (18 percent GLA), and spirulina.

Dihomo-gamma-linolenic acid (DGLA) is a derivative of GLA, but the only known direct source is mother's milk. It contributes to the protection of arteries and the heart, stimulates immunity, and has an anti-inflammatory effect.

Finally, arachidonic acid (AA) is a derivative of DGLA. Egg yolks and animal fats are its direct sources. AA assures the scarring and healing of wounds and contributes to the mechanisms of allergic reac-tions. Consumed in excess, it can provoke diseases like arthritis, eczema, psoriasis, and a number of autoimmune diseases.

What dose of omega-6 is necessary?

There is usually no need for omega-6 supplementation. We get ample amounts of omega-6s through our diet. Very seldom does someone need to supplement with omega-6s, and this is determined by a blood test.

How do you go about prescribing fatty acids?

I get to know my patients' needs through clinical examination and by questioning them about their lifestyle, eating habits, and their medical problems. If they agree, I suggest measuring the FAs in their cell membranes (with an erythrocyte membrane fatty acid test) in order to better understand any deficits and rebalancing that must be carried out. Advising an oil for use in the diet poses no problem, but a food supplement specifically containing omega-3s or omega-6s is more delicate. You cannot guess the correct amount, because their actions interrelate. A balance between omega-3s and omega-6s is essential to vitality.

What balance should we achieve between omega-3s and omega-6s?

Up until the 1920s, the production of edible oils was on a small scale. The oils were cold-pressed and sold in small quantities because they didn't keep for long. Indeed, the omega-3 FAs quickly went rancid when they were exposed to oxygen and light. The imperative for mass food production pushed the industry to favor oils that were more stable and therefore less rich in omega-3s, and to greatly refine the oils, which diminished still further their omega-3 content. What is more, the consumption of fish diminished, while the consumption of processed foods rich in omega-6s increased, and intensive agricultural and livestock farming techniques reduced the content of omega-3s in many foods, such as leafy green vegetables, meat, eggs, and even fish.

As a result, we estimate that, in general, the ratio between omega-6s and omega-3s in the Western diet is between 10:1 and 30:1, whereas it should ideally be between 1:1 and 4:1. What aggravates the situation is that this excess of omega-6 prevents the optimal use of omega-3 by the body, because they are in competition with each other! In fact, the metabolism of the omega-3s and omega-6s calls on the same enzymes and, in a modest way, on several of the same vitamins (vitamin B_3, B_6, C, and E) and minerals (magnesium and zinc). Excess omega-6s in our food, therefore, prevents the body from adequately exploiting the sources of omega-3.

This imbalance leads to, among other things, a physiological condition that favors cardiovascular disease as well as allergic and inflammatory problems. To top it all off, if a disease harms fatty acid metabolism, the problem is accentuated. Diabetes, as well as excess alcohol, tobacco, and stress can make it difficult or impossible for ALA to be transformed into EPA.

According to several experts, a return to food that provides an adequate ratio of omega-6s and omega-3s would have a positive effect on the cardiovascular health of the Western world and would also reduce inflammatory diseases.

What sort of problems are fatty acids good for?

Fatty acids are of real benefit to people confronting loss of memory, cardiovascular accidents, or accentuated dryness of the skin. They can also benefit those who are overweight: it has been noted that by making the cell membranes supple and facilitating nutrient exchanges and blood circulation, omega-3 helps to unload fat (a new way to control weight loss). Fatty acids also act against chronic inflammatory diseases through substances called prostaglandins types I and III, which are anti-inflammatory and protect the cell membranes.

What is your advice concerning dietary options for getting the right fatty acids?

Of foods, I especially recommend the use of flaxseed oil for seasoning. When it is of biological origin, conditioned in a tinted glass bottle, and kept in a cool place, flaxseed oil contains precursors of omega-3 fatty acids. We will abandon soy oil and walnut oil because of their high content of omega-6 FAs, which interfere with the omega-3 family. I advise using canola oil, which is richer in omega-3s, or flaxseed oil, which should not be heated.

Oily fish, such as Atlantic halibut, herring, sea trout, salmon, tuna, sardines, and mackerel, are also excellent sources of omega-3s. Oily fish should be eaten three or four times a week, raw or lightly cooked—quickly fried on each side, poached in water with the heat turned off, or marinated in lemon juice—because that way you preserve the fragile omega-3s. For those who prefer to avoid fish, I advise fish oil capsules. Here again, pay attention to the quality of the products you buy because these very fragile FAs will not support being exposed to heat and oxygen, or sitting on store shelves for too long.

My father was intuitive about the nutritional value of oily fish: he used to go fishing in his spare time and when he brought back trout the color of salmon, they were given to the children first. When we asked why, he simply replied, "Because they are the ones that are best for you." Where he had "fished" this information from—he was a photographer and knew nothing about biology—I'll never know. It was his instinct, or perhaps advice he got from his father, who already knew that trout that were like salmon were excellent for health.

My appreciation for fish probably started thirty years later in Lozere, France, at Marvejols, the royal town where Henry IV lived. I met a Chinese friend from Hong Kong, Ambrous, who told me an unusual story. When he was out cruising the waters off Alaska, the sailors caught an enormous fish weighing several hundred pounds, enough to feed the entire yacht for several weeks. He was surprised to note that, after four days of exclusively eating this Alaskan variety of fish, they were rejuvenated, with more vitality, more tonicity, and more sex drive. In short, this was an extraordinary experience for them.

It took me forty years to complete the picture and put together this nutritional program that is in part built on the experiences of my father and my Chinese friend. Thanks to both of them. Today, it's up to you to take advantage.

You recommended fish oil capsules for people who don't like to eat fish. Are there still other ways to obtain omega-3s?

If you don't like fish or you can't eat it often, do not despair—there are many delicious ways of increasing the content of omega-3 fatty acids in your diet. Here are some alternatives:

- Try to find eggs and meat that are rich in omega-3s. Some egg producers now use for feed a form of lettuce that has been enriched with omega-3 FAs, fish meal, or flaxseeds (and sometimes extra vitamin E). Chickens that eat this lettuce produce eggs with extra omega-3s.

- Choose meats and milk products from free-range animals fed on grass and insects (rather than those fattened up with seeds rich in omega-6s).

- When possible, eat game—it has fatty acids that closely resemble the FAs of the wild meats that our ancestors used to eat.

- Seek out other foods enriched with omega-3s, such as pasta sauces.

- If you don't like oily fish or any of the other foods suggested here, take supplements of seed oils containing omega-3s. The supplements should also contain vitamin E to prevent rancidity.

What are the beneficial effects of fish oil?

By taking fish oil—1,800 mg of eicosapentaenoic acid (EPA) and 1,200 mg of docosahexaenoic acid (DHA) per day for six weeks—we see an improvement in physical performance. Fish oil reduces bad cholesterol while encouraging an increase in good cholesterol. It also reduces high blood pressure and the risk of thromboembolic accident (obstruction of blood vessels), coronary stenosis (narrowing of coronary arteries), and cardiac rhythm problems. Fish oil diminishes the severity of rheumatic crises, inflammatory arthritis, and rheumatoid polyarthritis. And it reduces the risk of recurrence of inflammatory intestinal diseases, especially Crohn's disease.

Do fatty acids have a direct effect on cardiac arrhythmia?

Italian researchers have shown that in patients who have just suffered a myocardial infarction (heart attack), a low-dose supplement of omega-3 FAs reduces the risk of mortality and sudden death provoked by loss of cardiac rhythm. This study followed 11,323 patients who had suffered a myocardial infarction within the previous three months. They were randomly allocated fatty acids (1 gram per day of omega-3s), vitamin E (400 IU per day), both of them, or a placebo. After three months, mortality had significantly reduced in the group receiving omega-3s compared to the other groups. The reduction in the number of sudden deaths was marked after four months, and similar results were noted after six and eight months, concerning deaths of cardiovascular, cardiac, and coronary origin.

OILS RICH IN OMEGA-3S AND OMEGA-6S

The ratio of omega-6s to omega-3s in the Western diet is at least 10:1 instead of 4:1 or even 1:1 as it should be, because many of our foods are imbalanced with too many omega-6s. We, therefore, need to increase our consumption of omega-3 fatty acids. The omega-6 oils listed below are healthier than other choices but they should still be used in moderation to protect a healthy omega-6 to omega-3 ratio.

All of these products, with the exception of capelin oil, are to be kept strictly away from the light, heat, and damp. Also, it is imperative not to cook with them.

- The oil of squash seeds *(Cucurbita pepo)* is useful in treating prostate problems. It contains 50 percent linoleic acid (LA), an omega-6 fatty acid, and 12 percent of alpha-linolenic acid (ALA), an omega-3.

- Oil of capelin is taken from this fish (omega-3 series), which lives in the cold waters of Iceland. It is a good source of omega-3s, is very stable, and helps protect the blood vessels.

- Oil of cameline comes from a cruciferous plant *(Camelina sativa)*, which belongs to the family of oleaginous European plants. Its richness in alpha-linolenic acid (30 to 42 percent) from the omega-3 FAs is exceptional, which makes it resemble flaxseed oil and purslane (a plant that grows on poor, dry soil and is eaten in salads). It also contains omega-6s in good proportions (16 to 25 percent).

- Flaxseed oil is obtained from fresh, mature seeds. It is very rich in alpha-linolenic acid. It has an anticoagulant action and protects the cardiovascular system.

- Evening primrose oil contains 80 percent polyunsaturated fatty acids, of which 10 percent is gamma-linolenic acid (GLA), an omega-6 FA. It is recommended against excess cholesterol and has a favorable effect on premenstrual syndrome. Evening primrose oil also has an anticoagulant action and is useful for cardiovascular protection.

- Borage oil is obtained from borage seeds *(Borago officinalis)*. Its richness in gamma-linolenic acid (an omega-6 FA) makes it useful for treating premenstrual tension, menstrual pain, and inflammation. Some people also recommend it for irritability and depression.

- Carthame oil is extracted from the safflower seeds *(Carthamus tinctorius)* and contains at least 70 percent linoleic acid (LA), an omega-6. It can be served with mayonnaise, in salads, and in all kinds of seasonings. Because of the high omega-6 content, carthame oil should be used in moderation.

Researchers think that omega-3 FAs prevent cardiac arrhythmia, which is, in most cases, responsible for sudden death, and that they could provide an effective therapy. Be careful, though, as there can be interactions between omega-3s and anticoagulants and medicines for diabetes. You need to talk to your doctor before supplementing with omega-3s.

What oils do you recommend for eating?

Olive and canola oils are the best for eating, complemented by evening primrose, borage, camelina, and fish oils. They are all good for your health.

Only the virgin oils—first cold-pressing, which are obtained by simply pressing the fruit without adding solvents and without increasing the temperature—have a perfume, a color, a fruitiness, a fluidity, and a lightness that means they can be distinguished from one another. These nuances come from their composition of fatty acids, which are to oils what pigments are to colors—the base elements. Each fatty acid contains properties that deserve to be tasted and appreciated.

CHAPTER 9

Atherosclerosis and Arteriosclerosis

JULIEN: *Arteries and the cardiovascular system have been mentioned several times in our discussions, but we haven't talked about them directly. Now, don't they say that you are only as old as your arteries?*

DR. CHAUCHARD: Exactly. That's a popular expression and it's also a medical reality. Two aging factors are involved: atherosclerosis and arteriosclerosis, which are nothing more or less than inflammatory reactions of the arterial vessels.

Arterial vessels transport the blood throughout the body. Traveling to even the tiniest corner of the body, the blood brings the nutrients we need to live and takes away the waste that we need to eliminate. The engorgement of tissue from atherosclerosis and arteriosclerosis gradually brings about an asphyxia (lack of oxygen) of the entire cell system, while the sudden and brutal sealing up of the blood vessels gives rise to serious and sometimes fatal cardiovascular diseases. It is, therefore, vital that we keep our arteries healthy and thereby allow the agent that liaises between the vital functions—the blood—to accomplish its oxygenation function.

What is the difference between atherosclerosis and arteriosclerosis?

In general, the term *sclerosis* designates any fibrous degeneration of the tissue or organ. With age, the tissues that make up the arteries lose their elasticity and become more rigid. This normal aging of the arteries is called arteriosclerosis.

Arteriosclerosis is very often accompanied by fatty deposits (cholesterol) on the internal wall of the arteries. These whitish patches are called atheromas (from the Greek word *athere* meaning "gruel," which the fatty deposits were thought to resemble). Atherosclerosis, then, is when arteriosclerosis is accompanied by atheromas. Atherosclerosis involves the thickening of the wall of the large arteries (abdominal aorta, coronary, brain arteries, leg arteries) and their obstruction by atheromas.

Cholesterol is one of the fats that is transported by the blood. In excess, it is responsible for the formation of atheromas. This process resembles the way bathtub drains get coated with limestone. Over the years, these arterial deposits gradually become impregnated with fibrinogen, platelets, blood cells, and calcium, and then solidify.

What are the factors that lead to atherosclerosis?

A number of elements are likely to favor the onset and aggravation of atherosclerosis:

- *Lifestyle*—smoking, obesity, stress, sedentary habits, oral contraception, and alcoholism
- *Genetic factors*—family antecedents of cardiovascular accidents
- *Metabolic pathologies*—excess cholesterol, diabetes, and gout
- *High blood pressure*

What are the risks of smoking?

Nicotine encourages the brusque shrinking of the arteries (spasms). Smoke diminishes the supply of oxygen to the tissues and keeps an excessive level of carbon dioxide in the blood.

For those who smoke more than ten cigarettes per day, the risks are considerable. Addiction to tobacco multiplies by three the risk of a myocardial infarction (heart attack). For those smoking more than twenty cigarettes per day, the risk of heart attack is multiplied by five and risk of sudden death increases sixfold. Stopping smoking reduces vascular mortality by 50 percent.

What about stress?

Stress frees up adrenaline, which provokes spasms in the arteries. When stress is repeated too often, or is chronic, it can bring on high blood pressure and repeated arterial spasms that "use up" the arterial system and encourage atherosclerosis.

Why should we avoid being too sedentary?

Lack of physical activity reduces the resistance of the arteries, while exercise increases the level of "good cholesterol." Walking, swimming, and jogging seem to be the most effective sports to prevent or slow down the evolution of atherosclerosis.

Is it true that birth control pills and menopause are aggravating factors?

Yes. Oral contraception (the Pill) and menopause (especially when it is early) are risk factors in atherosclerosis. Atherosclerosis is caused by inflammation of the inner wall of the blood vessel (oxidative stress). The Pill is made from a synthetic estrogen, which when taken in high dosage causes inflammation of the vessel wall. Menopause is when the body's natural estrogen falls drastically—this, again, causes oxidative stress to the vessel wall, resulting in atherosclerosis. In the absence of an associated risk factor (including tobacco use), and combined with a diet that is low in saturated fats, the Pill can nevertheless be pre-scribed up to a total cholesterol level of 3 grams per liter (7.7 mmol/l). Low-dose oral contraception is recommended and the patient must be closely monitored.

What is the effect of high cholesterol?

There is a direct link between food that is rich in animal fats and ath-erosclerosis. The development of atheromas on the artery walls is linked to an increase of fats in the blood, and especially oxidized cho-lesterol. LDL (low-density lipoprotein) cholesterol—the "bad" cholesterol that causes most of the damage to the blood vessel walls—is produced in the liver. Dietary cholesterol will raise the total cholesterol level, which is still harmful for the vessel wall but not as bad as high LDL cholesterol.

Do genetic factors play a part?

It is sometimes difficult to distinguish between real heredity and habits linked to lifestyle. In any case, we know that genetic history plays a part in a predisposition to atherosclerosis. Hereditary factors are well-established: 30 percent of men with coronary disease had fathers who died of coronary disease. Being a man makes you more vulnerable to the disease, but this difference between men and women diminishes after menopause. Furthermore, high cholesterol that runs in the family is the most frequent of all genetic diseases.

What are the symptoms?

The development of cardiovascular lesions is progressive and problems appear about the age of forty or fifty, maybe even older, when the critical level of artery obstruction is achieved (70 to 80 percent) and the cells of the organs (heart, brain, kidneys, muscles) start to lack oxygen. The symptoms presented by a patient suffering from atherosclerosis entirely depend on which arteries are affected. Symptoms are as follows:

- *Coronary arteries*—angina and myocardial infarction (heart attack)
- *Cerebral arteries*—cerebral vascular accidents due to the obstruction of one or several arteries that feed the brain
- *Aorta*—aortic aneurysm, aortic dissection
- *Arteries of the lower limbs*—arteritis obstructing blood flow to the lower limbs
- *Renal (kidney) arteries*—high pressure in the renal arteries

Is there a link between high blood pressure and atherosclerosis?

Whatever its origin, high blood pressure provokes or aggravates atherosclerosis, and vice versa, atherosclerosis complicates and aggravates high blood pressure.

How can you identify atherosclerosis?

The three key moments in examining a patient suffering from atherosclerosis are as follows:

1. The interview, which takes into account all the risk factors presented by the patient.

2. Taking the patient's blood pressure in a seated position after the patient has rested calmly for ten to fifteen minutes.

3. Feeling the pulse in the neck, the groin (femoral artery), and the feet.

This basic examination can be followed by listening to the superficial arterial courses in search of a murmur, as proof of arterial shrinkage. Only the large arteries whose courses are not too deep are accessible for direct clinical examination: the aorta, carotids, femoral, and leg arteries. The Doppler scan, which visualizes the interior of the vessels, is an easy and excellent test that is almost obligatory.

Finally, we proceed with a biological blood test, which determines blood levels of cholesterol, triglycerides, glucose, glycosyl hemoglobin, and uric acid. Normal levels are as follows:

Normal total cholesterol level

- Aged under thirty: 1.55–1.80 gram/liter (4.0–5.2 millimoles/liter)
- Aged over thirty: 1.8–2.0 g/l (5.2–6.4 mmol/l)

Normal level of HDL ("good") cholesterol

- Men: 0.4–0.65 g/l (1.0–1.65 mmol/l)
- Women: 0.5–0.8 g/l (1.3–2.0 mmol/l)

Normal level of LDL ("bad") cholesterol

- Men: 1.1–1.6 g/l (2.84–4.13 mmol/l)
- Women: 1.0–1.5 g/l (2.58–3.87 mmol/l)

Normal level of triglycerides

- Men: 0.5–1.5 g/l (0.6–1.7 mmol/l)
- Women: 0.4–1.3 g/l (0.45–1.50 mmol/l)

Normal level of glycemia

- On an empty stomach: 0.70–1.0 g/l (3.9–5.6 mmol/l)
- Two hours after a meal: less than 1.20 g/l (less than 6.7 mmol/l)

Normal levels of glycosyl hemoglobin

- HbA1a + HbA1b: 6 to 8 percent
- HbA1c: 4 to 6 percent

Normal levels of uric acid

- Men: 30–70 milligrams/liter (180–420 mmol/l)
- Women: 20–60 mg/l (60–210 mmol/l)

A biological hormonal assessment can be requested in the light of the results of the clinical and biological examinations. The following tests are never systematically requested in the course of a basic assessment, but only if the clinical signs suggest the effects of athero-sclerosis on a particular organ (the target organ):

- Electrocardiogram while at rest (and sometimes during physical effort)

- Carotid, coronary, or renal arteriography

What are the complications of atherosclerosis?

One complication of atherosclerosis occurs when the artery becomes totally blocked (thrombosis), impeding circulation to the area, causing tissue death.

Also, the blood clot that forms around the atheroma patch is some-times crumbly. Part of it might become detached and move further on in the artery. When this clot stops in a smaller artery, it creates an embolism.

How can we prevent atherosclerosis? And what can we do to treat it?

Above all, it is a fight against risk factors. Good food, aspirin (acetylsalicylic acid), and omega-3 fatty acids are the basic treatment. If the person is obese or overweight, then follow my 30-Day Timely Nutrition Vitality Program (see Chapter 10), based on good lipids, good carbohydrates, and little alcohol (once again, an insulin-resistance treatment).

If the person is not obese, he or she can follow a diet that is low in saturated animal fats and fast-acting, refined carbohydrates (those with a high glycemic index). Today, we consume on average 600 milligrams of cholesterol per day, whereas 300 milligrams should be the limit.

For preventing or treating atherosclerosis, it's a good idea to do the following:

- Consume polyunsaturated and monounsaturated vegetable fats (sunflower, corn, canola, olive, and grapeseed oils).

- Avoid fats of animal origin (except at breakfast) and saturated fats (such as whole milk).

- Avoid food that is rich in cholesterol: egg yolk, organ meats, walnuts, almonds, cream, lobster, shellfish, and fish eggs (including caviar).

- Eat plenty of fish, veal, and chicken, and drink very little alcohol.

- Eat garlic. Garlic keeps the blood fluid through the action of one of its component parts, ajoene, which inhibits blood aggregation (although watch out for allergies and bad breath).

WINE AND YOUR HEART

The moderate consumption of wine has a protective effect on the arteries. But be careful: excess alcohol plays a role in high blood pressure and can lead to addiction and alcoholism. Only drink wine with meals, rather than before or after meals.

- When diet is not enough to bring the cholesterol level back to normal, cholesterol-lowering medications may be prescribed: fibrates, statins, and cholestyramines are the most common.

- When only the triglyceride level is high and if diet and cutting out alcohol are not sufficient to bring it down, fibrates, fish oils, or vegetable oils based on flaxseed (rich in polyunsaturated omega-3 FAs) are recommended.

The rest of the treatment consists of fighting against high blood pressure (using diet with or without blood-pressure-lowering drugs) and smoking (stopping smoking makes the increased vascular risk disappear in five years).

Finally, if you follow my 30-day nutrition program, your cardiovascular risks will very quickly disappear, because the heart and the vessels regenerate even before your skin and general health does. We will discuss my nutrition program in detail in the next chapter.

CHAPTER 10

The 30-Day Timely Nutrition Vitality Program

B y reading this book, you are educating yourself about nutrition. Knowing what different foods are made of and how they affect the body is an important start to reclaiming your vitality. Adhering to my method works, because those who follow it understand the food choices they are making, instead of mindlessly sticking to ready-made menus.

In terms of diet, there are still some commonly held misconceptions about what is healthy that we need to get rid of. For instance, the low-calorie diet has proved inefficient for long-term health, so there is no longer any point in recommending it. Rather than reinforcing notions that have become outdated, we should take into account recent scientific work. My program incorporates the new knowledge we have of "timely nutrition": we eat what our body needs, according to our daily activities and, above all, according to the digestive secretions of each organ involved in the digestive process.

My program is anti-inflammatory, antioxidant, and anti-glycation; it restructures your body and returns it to its proper condition. For thirty years, ever since I was a young doctor, I have been looking for an ideal nutritional model that is easy to follow, not restrictive, and convivial— in other words, one that is pleasant and allows you to eat everything. Was that like trying to square a circle? In fact, I needed all that time to put together this 30-Day Timely Nutrition Vitality Program. It is "timely" because we need to eat in concert with the body's organs. "Nutrition" refers to a good choice of foods, as opposed to dieting or calorie restriction. It is a 30-day program because after thirty days of food regulation it is much easier to control the body: in that amount of time the body's insulin secretion drops and the immune system becomes more stable. It is the ideal program because all the patients who have followed it accept the guidelines easily and judge it an ideal lifetime nutrition program, where "lifetime" really does mean for the rest of your life. In other words, this is a nutrition concept to integrate into our everyday lives, and for always.

LEARN TO BE IN CONTROL OF YOUR WEIGHT WITH "TIMELY NUTRITION"

Each of the five essential organs is more or less active in terms of digestive secretion at each moment of the day. This timely nutrition method allows you to reduce the burden of weight wherever you need to. It then ensures a long-term stabilization of your weight that can last forever if you stick with my concept. The five organs involved in digestion are the brain, liver, stomach, pancreas, and the kidneys.

Morning

Let us call the brain the "chief organizer" who controls the "call to eat." As soon as we wake up in the morning we need the energy that fat, in general, brings; we need protein to synthesize new cells; and we need a certain amount of starch so that the energy combustion process occurs in optimal conditions. The liver is necessary because its secretions do their best to digest the fat and organize the synthesis of protein. The stomach is also always available—it doesn't really have a choice in the matter!

In the morning, sugars rapidly absorbed by the body should be avoided, as we do not want to encourage secretions from the pancreas at this time. The right moment for sugar will be in the afternoon, when the pancreas will naturally produce an insulin peak and the body can receive sugar without biological damage. That way we avoid producing excess insulin and, thereby, do not end up with insulin resistance.

Midday

At lunchtime, we need proteins—red or white meat or fish—a small helping of starch, and 250 grams of non-starchy green vegetables. Add to that a little olive oil to hold it all together and to avoid hunger.

Afternoon

An afternoon snack is permitted on the program. The pancreas produces insulin to put the blood glucose into cells or divert it to fat. According to the effective times and functions of our organs, the natural peak insulin secretion is in the afternoon, around 4 to 6 P.M. So, eating fruit plus a slice of dark chocolate (70 percent cocoa) at this time causes no harm to the body.

Evening

At the end of the day, the liver and its digestive secretions are at a minimum, so no more animal fat at this time, except good fats in the form of olive oil and oily fish. You should, above all, avoid soliciting the services of the pancreas—not a trace of sugar, starch, alcohol, or fruit. In the evening, the pancreas is on holiday, sleeping and resting. Ideally, only the stomach is working at night, in addition to the kidneys, which must then start cleansing the body. We say that the kidneys do the washing up during the night.

A good night's cleansing means you wake up happy, without the bad mood that comes with a heavy tongue. Whenever it is difficult to wake up, it is due to a complicated nocturnal digestion, with too many different sorts of food, too much alcohol, too much sugar and fat. We are talking about a digestive cacophony provoking significant disruption.

All those with fat around the stomach can practically lose it all simply by respecting an evening meal as I have just described—oily fish or any fish, non-starchy vegetables, and nothing else.

A GLOBAL APPROACH TO LIVING BETTER

This program is not confined to losing weight: it's a preventive, whole-body approach aimed at improving overall health and quality of life for the long-term. In other words, it is a global approach to living better.

You will not only look and feel better, but you will concurrently diminish or eradicate problems such as stress and cardiovascular risk. Stress encourages inflammatory reactions by secreting the hormones such as cortisol. This program improves your health and your skin, helps you to burn up fat, and thus relieves your stress. Additionally, a diet rich in vitamins, trace elements, and mineral salts will allow you to reclaim all your vitality. Choosing the right fats and carbohydrates, as well as enriching the diet with fibers and antioxidants, allows you to reduce cardiovascular risk.

This program should help you to better understand your relationship with food and discover that eating less and slimming down can also be a source of pleasure. Above all, eating must remain a convivial act, a source of pleasure. My method proves that weight loss and rejuvenation are not synonymous with sad meals or deprivation. You can eat what you like at the right time of day. Tell me what you like to eat, I'll tell you when you can eat your favorite food.

THE TIMELY NUTRITION VITALITY PROGRAM

Now that you understand the basic principles behind the 30-Day Timely Nutrition Vitality Program, you are ready for the program itself. In this section I outline fifteen "golden rules," give you healthy food combinations, and tell you what times of day are appropriate to eat given foods. I then recommend high-quality foods to choose from and cooking methods to use, provide you with a sample daily menu, and suggest appropriate consumption levels. After following this program for thirty days, you will find that you have more control over your body and that you feel and look better and younger.

The Golden Rules

Use these fifteen rules as your guide throughout the program. They serve as your ticket to increased vitality and the backbone of the daily menu presented later in the chapter.

1. Start all your meals with protein—proteins above all! You can use the following formula* to calculate your protein ration yourself:
   - Portion of red meat in grams: add 100 to your height in centimeters. (Example: 170 centimeters + 100 = 270 grams of meat.)
   - Portion of white meat in grams: subtract 40 from your height in centimeters. (Example: 170 centimeters − 40 = 130 grams of roast chicken or turkey.)

2. Drink more water. Here is a formula* to determine the appropriate amount of water (in liters) to keep your body healthy, add your height in centimeters plus your weight in kilograms, then divide by 100. For example, if you measure 1.70 meters high and weigh 70 kilograms, it will be (170 + 70) ÷ 100 = 2.4 liters of water per day, every day (and more when the weather is hot).
   - Drink a glass of water (at room temperature) as soon as you wake up.
   - Drink another glass before breakfast.
   - Drink a glass of water roughly every hour.

   If you don't drink water, you cannot metabolize fat, nor can your body get rid of the cells' waste. A dehydrated body encourages aging and inflammatory reactions.

3. Have three meals a day, plus a snack between 4 and 5 P.M.

4. If you find yourself hungry during the day, eat more protein and increase your ration of olive oil.

5. Above all, avoid foods that stimulate the pancreas and provoke insulin excess, such as coffee, fast food, and sugary foods (see "Foods to Avoid" on page 107).

---

*Metric measurements are required for this formula. A conversion chart can help you figure your height in centimeters and weight in kilograms, if necessary.

6. Eat more fish, especially oily fish such as organic salmon (see "Our Favorite Fish" on page 106).

7. Avoid sugary foods whenever possible. If you need something sweet, eat it only between 4 and 5 P.M. For example, eat a bar of dark chocolate with at least 70 percent cocoa (you can now find chocolate with up to 86 percent cocoa), plus a piece of fruit (choose from the list of recommended fruits).

8. At dinner, no starch is allowed or fried foods. Eat your ration of vegetables and no more.

9. Choose your fruit according to the recommended list and eat it at the correct time for proper absorption, either late morning or during the afternoon.

10. Eat more slowly—food should be almost liquid before you swallow it!

11. If you're not hungry in the evening, eat less or skip dinner.

12. Never forget olive oil and lemon juice to taste.

13. Choose good fats, like olive oil or avocado or oily fish, and avoid bad fats that destroy the cell membranes (especially fried animal fat). Your cell membranes are as important as your legs—these membranes are the legs of your cells.

14. Take all your food supplements with your meals. Remember, don't drink anything hot after taking omega-3 and omega-6 supplements.

15. You are allowed one or two "wild cards" per week—no more—to deviate from the program. Use these wild cards when you have no other option, and eat your favorite food. Only one wild card is permitted if your aim is to lose weight.

Food Groupings and Timely Combinations

Group 1 and group 2 foods can be eaten anytime; group 3 fats should be eaten at meals according to the Food Combinations Schedule;

group 4 foods should be eaten only in the morning and at lunch; and group 5 vegetables can be eaten anytime (fruit should be eaten outside mealtimes, preferably in the afternoon).

Group 1: Proteins

- Meat (with skin removed)—beef, chicken, fowl, lamb, pork, turkey, veal

- Fish—oily varieties (see "Our Favorite Fish" on page 106)

- Shellfish—clams, crabs, crawfish, lobsters, mussels, octopus, oysters, prawns, scallops, shrimps, snails

Group 2: Other Proteins

- Milk—skim or part-skim; yogurt

- Cheese—brie, Camembert, cottage cheese, feta, goat's cheese, low-fat cheese, mozzarella, Muenster, Parmesan, Romano, Roquefort (*Note: Those who don't like cheese must take a supplement of calcium with vitamin D in the evening.*)

- Eggs

Group 3: Fats (Lipids)

- Oils—canola oil, grapeseed oil, flaxseed oil, olive oil, sesame oil, sunflower oil

- Nuts—almonds, Brazil nuts, cashews, chestnuts, pecans, pine nuts, pistachios

---

FOOD COMBINATIONS SCHEDULE

Breakfast: protein (group 1) + carbohydrates (group 4) + fat (group 3)

Lunch: protein (group 1) + carbohydrates (group 4)

Afternoon: carbohydrates (group 4) + vegetable or fruit fat (group 3)

Dinner: protein (fish or white meat) + non-starchy vegetables

---

- Fruit high in fat such as avocado and durian

Group 4: Slowly Absorbed Carbohydrates

- Grains—rice (except white rice), pasta (choose whole-wheat pasta), bread (except white bread), oatmeal, barley

- Legumes

- Starchy vegetables such as potatoes

Group 5: Ultra-Slowly Absorbed Carbohydrates

- Non-starchy vegetables (see "Recommended Vegetables" below)

- Fruits—apples, apricots, berries, cherries, citrus fruits, melons (except watermelon), peaches, pears, plums

Recommended Foods

The following lists of recommended foods offer a wide variety of high-quality choices to keep meals nutritional and interesting. Add foods to the diet according to the Food Combinations Schedule.

Recommended Vegetables

Asparagus	Leafy vegetables
Broccoli	Lettuce (all forms)
Brussels sprouts	Mushrooms
Cabbage (green, red, or Chinese)	Onions
Cauliflower	Peppers (any color, sweet and hot)
Celery	Spinach
Chicory	Summer squash
Cucumbers	Tomatoes
Eggplant	Vegetables with roots
Green or yellow beans	Zucchini

Recommended Fruits

Apples

Apricots

Avocados

Berries (blackberries, blueberries,
raspberries, strawberries)

Cherries

Citrus fruits (grapefruits, oranges,
lemons)

Grapes

Melons (except watermelon)

Peaches

Pears

Persimmon

Plums

Rhubarb

THE SEVEN FAMILIES OF VEGETABLES AND FRUITS

Red—Rich in lycopene (a good antioxidant for protecting the prostate). Tomatoes belong to this family; only watermelon should be
avoided.

Purple—Rich in anthocyan (a good antioxidant for protecting the
heart and the brain). Strawberries, black currants, blackberries, plums,
apples, and green pepper all belong to this family.

Orange/Yellow—Rich in beta-cryptoxanthin (a good antioxidant for
transferring messages to the cells) and, of course, rich in vitamin C.
In this family, choose only oranges or peaches.

Pure Orange—Rich in vitamin A and good for the skin. This family
should be avoided except for raw carrots and melon.

White/Green—Rich in antitumor factors and antioxidants. Garlic, parsley, basil, celery, chicory, and pear are recommended; but limit grapes.

Yellow/Green—Rich in lutein and the carotenoid zeaxanthin (good
antioxidants and good for the eyes). Little beans, spinach, pears, avocados, and melon belong to this family.

Green—Rich in antioxidants, vitamins A, C, and E, and products that
destroy certain cancerous cells, principally in the lungs and the
colon. These include broccoli, green cabbage, Chinese cabbage, and
Brussels sprouts.

Recommended Meats

Beef	Fowl	Veal
Chicken	Turkey	

Recommended Legumes

Black beans	Lentils	Pinto beans
Chickpeas	Lima beans	Soybeans
Kidney beans		

Recommended Grains

Barley (whole, for soups)   Oatmeal (traditionally cooked)

OUR FAVORITE FISH

In general, the higher the level of fat in a fish, the higher its level of omega-3 fatty acids, which are good for our cell membranes.

FISH WITH A HIGH LEVEL OF POLYUNSATURATED FATS (MORE THAN 5 PERCENT FAT)

- Anchovies (unsalted, fresh)
- Capelin
- Eel
- Fresh herring
- John Dory
- Mackerel
- Red mullet
- Salmon (the pinker, the better; choose Alaskan or organic salmon)
- Sardines
- Trout (the pinker, the better)
- Tuna

FISH WITH AN AVERAGE FAT CONTENT (2.5 TO 5 PERCENT FAT)

- Atlantic halibut
- Swordfish
- Mullet

FISH WITH A LOW FAT CONTENT (LESS THAN 2.5 PERCENT FAT)

- Bass
- Cod
- Haddock (fresh)
- Hake
- Gudgeon
- Lingcod
- Pacific halibut
- Red snapper
- Shark
- Sole

Recommended Condiments

Extra-virgin olive oil   Mustard

Recommended Frozen Foods

Those guaranteed free from additives and artificial colors

Recommended Beverages

Herbal tea
Spring or mineral water (tap water is also quite acceptable)
Tea (all forms)

Recommended Herbs and Spices

Aniseed	Cumin	Oregano
Basil	Dried red pepper	Paprika
Bay leaves	Garlic	Rosemary
Cinnamon	Ginger (fresh)	Thyme
Coriander	Mint	

Foods to Avoid

These foods dramatically stimulate the pancreas to release insulin. They should, therefore, be completely avoided during the program.

Alcoholic drinks (including aperitifs, strong alcohol, beer, and liqueurs)

Bacon

Bananas

Butter

Cakes

Cookies

Cereals (except whole-grain varieties)

Chocolate (except chocolate containing at least 70 percent cocoa)

Coffee

Cream

Croissants (except at 4 P.M. for those who don't have weight to lose)

Dried fruits

Fast food

Foods with excessive animals fats

Fried food

Granola

Hard cheese (except feta, parmesan, and Romano)

Hot dogs

Ice cream

Jams and jellies

Mangoes

Margarine

Molasses

Muffins

Pancakes

Pastries

Peas

Pickles

Pizzas

Popcorn

Pudding

Pumpkin

Soft drinks (including commercial fruit juice)

Sorbet

Sponge cake

Sugar and sugary foods

Tacos

Tarts

Waffles

Recommended Cooking and Preparation Methods

Use the following cooking methods and food-preparation tips during the program to achieve optimal nutrition, vitality—and delicious meals.

- Marinate (in lemon juice and oil or wine for three to twenty-four hours) before cooking. Fatty fish are well suited for marination.

- Cook food slowly or keep food warm in a *bain-marie,* or Mary's bath (double saucepans, in which a smaller nonstick frying pan is set in a larger pan containing hot water).

- Gently fry food in a little vegetable juice or stock, without added oil.

- Poach fish in water with the heat turned off—either in a fish kettle, where the fish stock is brought to the boil and poured onto the fish, or in a saucepan sealed with a lid after turning off the heat as soon the water is simmering.

- Gently steam grains in a rice cooker or a couscous machine with a dome lid (to avoid droplets of water scalding the food).

- Cook legumes and cereals (except pasta) in a small amount of water, so all the water is absorbed once the food is cooked.

- In the oven, protect the food in an earthenware casserole dish.

- Cook food in a convection oven at low temperatures, 250–300°F.

- Prepare teas, infusions, and herbal teas with mineral water, without adding milk (which prevents the absorption of the protective elements in tea).

- Cook cereals and beans in mineral water.

- Cook cereals and ungerminated beans that are difficult to digest when raw. Otherwise, eat germinated cereals and beans raw.

- Always cook meats and eggs for hygienic reasons and to destroy anti-enzymes and anti-vitamins.

- Preferably use raw or lightly cooked fruit and vegetables.

- Cook potatoes whole in dry heat or steam with their skins on (if they are organic).

- Halve the quantity of sugar used in most recipes. Replace white sugar with organic brown sugar (containing molasses). Use in moderation honey and maple syrup, which are rich in glucose and fructose.

- Use unsweetened fruit purées instead of jam, replace sugary spreads with oily purées (almonds, hazelnuts), and replace ice cream with lightly sweetened sorbets.

- Use light sauces, such as a hollandaise sauce made from beaten egg whites and tomato sauce or carrot sauce.

- Keep oils away from the light. Flaxseed oil and evening primrose oil should be kept dry and away from the light, in the refrigerator, after opening.

- Use legumes, which are good sources of protein and fiber.

- Incorporate more soy-based products, obtained by extraction (soy milk, yogurt, and tofu) or by fermentation (tempura and miso).

- In a vegetarian meal, combine two sources of protein (for example, legumes and grains such as bulgur and whole-grain rice or pasta) in the same meal.

- Choose yogurts (containing the beneficial bacteria *Streptococcus thermophilus* and *Lactobacillus bulgaricus*) without added skim milk and made from goat's milk, sheep's milk, cow's milk, or soy milk.

- Use dairy products that are fermented and/or fermented soy products (containing healthy bacteria such as *Bifidobacterium, Lactobacillus casei, L. acidophilus, L. rhamnosus, Streptococcus lactis,* and *S. faecum*).

- Choose organic products (free from pesticides).

Cooking and Preparation Methods to Avoid

Be sure to steer clear of the following poor techniques and bad habits while cooking and preparing food.

- Avoid cooking food in the oven above 180°C/355°F, which causes the formation of toxic and carcinogenic products.

- Avoid horizontal barbecues, which lead to the formation of benzopyrene, a carcinogen. Instead, use a vertical barbeque.

- Avoid deep-frying, grilling, sealing, or browning food, especially meat and fish, which causes the formation of highly mutagenic products.

- Avoid cooking food in the pressure cooker or the microwave, which destroys all the vitamins.

- Avoid cooking food in aluminum pans (the aluminum transfers into the food).

- Avoid using the cooking juices of meat, which can contain toxic components.

- Don't add salt to your food. Remove the salt shaker from the table—we often add salt without thinking.

- Avoid canned food (bisphenol A is put into the food during sterilization)—favor fresh or frozen foods.

- Avoid roasted foods, except for fish and poultry whose skin is removed after cooking.

- Avoid products that have been cooked until brown: pastries, tart and quiche bases, cakes, and biscuits.

- Avoid peanut oil (rich in saturated fatty acids), hydrogenized margarine, and deep-frying oil.

- Avoid products using refined oil or hydrogenized margarine (rich in unhealthy fatty acids)—use non-hydrogenated margarine, preferably organic, and do not cook it.

A Daily Menu

The following daily menu provides suggested meals and snacks for the thirty days of the program. However, you should adapt the meals to add variety and to suit your tastes and lifestyle. By all means, experiment with different foods from the recommended lists. The important thing to remember is the proper association of proteins, fats, carbohydrates, vegetables, and fruits. The worst combination in the same meal is fast-burning carbohydrates and animal fats. Again, group 1 and group 2 foods (proteins) can be eaten anytime; group 3 (fats) should be eaten according to the food combinations schedule; group 4 foods (carbohydrates) should be eaten only in the morning and at lunch; and group 5 vegetables can be eaten anytime (fruit should be eaten outside mealtimes, preferably in the afternoon).

Upon Waking

Drink a large glass of water at room temperature. Have another glass of water or a cup of tea before breakfast.

Breakfast

- White omelette made with 3 egg whites plus 1 yolk, *or* 1 slice of skinless turkey, roast chicken, or unsmoked salmon

- 2.1–2.8 ounces bread

- 2.1–2.8 ounces cheese

- 1 or 2 tomatoes plus olive oil (essential)
- Unlimited tea

10 A.M.

1 cup of tea (your choice of tea)

11 A.M.

1 cup of tea, can be replaced by water

12 P.M.

1 cup of tea with or without a lemon slice

Lunch

- 8.75 ounces of fish from the recommended list (see "Our Favorite Fish" on page 106), especially salmon, *or* 8.75 ounces of red meat (twice a week) or white meat
- 1 cup of broccoli or other recommended vegetables plus olive oil and lemon juice
- Choice of starch: 1 small bowl of steamed rice, or whole-grain pasta (same quantity), or 1.75 ounces of whole-grain bread

3 P.M.

Green tea or water

4 P.M.

Green tea or water (in the afternoon, green tea is recommended because it doesn't disturb your sleep)

4–5 P.M.

- 1 bar of very dark chocolate (up to 86 percent cocoa is perfect; minimum of 70 percent cocoa)
- 1 piece of a recommended fruit or an avocado with olive oil

RECOMMENDED CONSUMPTION LEVELS

- *Fruit:* once or twice a day, including freshly squeezed juice (taken outside mealtimes, ideally at 11 A.M. and 4 P.M.)

- *Raw vegetables:* once a day

- *Green vegetables:* twice a day

- *Root vegetables:* 1–3 times a week

- *Cereals:* follow your doctor's advice

- *Slice of whole-grain bread or portion of whole-grain rice:* once or twice a day (breakfast and lunch)

- *Legumes:* once or twice a week

- *Soy in the form of milk or tofu:* 2–3 times a week

- *Oily nuts:* equivalent of five hazelnuts or almonds, 2–3 times a week

- *Oils rich in omega-3s (such as olive oil):* 1–2 tablespoons per day

- *Fish:* 6–7 times a week, including oily fish 3–4 times a week

- *Shellfish:* once or twice a week

- *Yogurt or other fermented dairy products:* follow the advice of your doctor (allowed at 11 A.M. or during the afternoon)

- *Eggs:* between 6 and 8 a week, according to the advice of your doctor

- *Poultry (meat and liver):* 2–3 times a week

- *Mineral or spring water:* 1.5 quarts per day, at least

- *Tea:* 1–3 cups per day

- *Wine:* up to one glass per day

If you are not at home, 10 hazelnuts or 10 almonds can replace the chocolate or avocado, followed by a recommended fruit.

6 P.M.

1 glass of water or cup of green tea

7 P.M.

1 glass of water or cup of green tea

Dinner

- Recommended oily fish (8.75 ounces at least), preferably salmon, tuna, or mackerel

- Recommended vegetables (1 cup)

  Note: I recommend putting olive oil on all appropriate foods.

"Long Life" Antioxidant Soup   YIELD: SIX SERVINGS

This is one of my favorite recipes. It is ideal for lunch or dinner.

6 large onions

2 green peppers

1 large cabbage

1 stalk of celery

1 tomato

1–2 8-ounce cans peeled or chopped tomatoes

spices to taste

*1 packet powdered soup mix
without noodles (optional)*

Cut the vegetables into medium-sized cubes and place in a saucepan with canned tomatoes. Add your favorite spices, spicy sauce, herbs, and so on. You can also add powdered soup. Cover with water and cook with the lid on for 45 minutes or until the vegetables are tender.

Tips for Success

Here are a few pieces of advice to help you achieve optimal success and vitality with the program: Don't eat before or after meals. If you are hungry, increase your proteins and olive oil. If you overeat, skip the next dinner. If you overindulge again, say over the weekend, on Monday follow the breakfast and 4 P.M. snack as prescribed, but eat only fish and vegetables for the other two meals. When you are invited out to dinner, you can limit the damage by concentrating on avoiding starch, sugar, desserts, or fruit.

Remember, you can adapt the Timely Nutrition Vitality Program to suit your lifestyle, and you should. The important thing is to maintain the proper association of proteins, fats, carbohydrates, vegetables, and fruits. After following the program for thirty days, your insulin levels will be lower and you will experience less inflammation. As a result, free-radical production will decline and the health and longevity of your cells will increase.

HANDLING YOUR STRESS TO AGE LESS QUICKLY

In addition to dietary changes, staying young and vibrant requires learning to handle the stresses of everyday life.

- Always think positively, think about longevity and *joie de vivre.*

- If you are stressed, whether it is physical or psychological, try not to have negative thoughts—think of your well-being and other pleasurable thoughts.

- Love life.

- Know how to be adaptable and accept change.

- Avoid a sedentary lifestyle.

- Love laughter.

- Take time to get to know yourself and become fulfilled.

- Learn to appreciate yourself—be tolerant of yourself and others, control your emotions, and don't react rashly.

- Accept happy and sad events as they happen and make the best of them.

- Don't look back, look forward!

- Find at least three things that give you satisfaction every day.

- Remain open to the sensual and spoil yourself regularly.

- Sometimes, be lazy and indulge in futile pleasures.

- Don't be unrealistic in your expectations—many frustrations are founded in utopian ideas of happiness.

- Whatever happens, take notes and share them with your doctor. He or she can help you solve your problems.

CHAPTER 11

The Journey to Outer Beauty

JULIEN: *Now that I have taken care of my "inside" and the overall balance of my body, what can I do for my outward appearance and, especially, how can I rejuvenate my face as swiftly as my body?*

DR. CHAUCHARD: First of all, what is good inside looks good outside. Everything we have spoken of, especially all the advice in terms of food, encourages a "healthy look" and a good complexion, prolonging the vitality of the skin and delaying aging.

Just as in the rest of this rejuvenation program, the aesthetic or outward aspect is a question of choice and will. Each of us has a particular relationship with our "exterior" aspect. We can live perfectly well with wrinkles, but the rejuvenation of the face can also be a catalyst for a global, or complete, rejuvenation of the body. If you feel good in yourself, you will be even more motivated to make the necessary effort to keep in shape. When you are in shape, your vitality increases, and so does your *joie de vivre*. It is what is known as a "virtuous circle." Personal radiance often shows in the face.

Just as it is legitimate to lift our features, to make ourselves look good, to efface the ravages on our necks, so it is pointless to try to "appear" twenty years younger, which will never be the case. An injection can repair the damage from a part of your life when you were not in control of our diet, physique, and sorrows. An injection can lift morale as well as physical form, and that is already a lot.

Natural (intrinsic) aging brings changes to the texture of the skin. With age, the skin becomes finer, dry, finely wrinkled, and loses its elasticity. Intrinsic aging is accompanied by a progressive degeneration of the structure and function of the skin. The proliferation of cells diminishes in the epidermis (outer skin layer) and in the lower skin tissues, in which the structural proteins are found. The skin's collagen and fibroblasts diminish. The blood irrigation, or microcirculation, is also reduced, leading to a slowing down in the scarring process. The mechanical resistance to trauma is also diminished.

All these combined effects gradually give the skin a dry, flaccid, and fragile appearance. The natural lines of the face, those famous character lines, programmed from birth, become deeper and more marked. The breaks in the elastin and collagen fibers generate other hollows, particularly around the mouth. Next come the first white hairs, the first little wrinkles, and bags beneath the eyes. Then appear wrinkles, age spots, and other evidence of encroaching old age.

Age spots, marks of hyperpigmentation, are due to the decreasing number and faulty functioning of our melanocytes (the cells that produce the pigment melanin). Brutal exposure to the sun, which must be avoided as soon as these marks begin to appear, can only increase the number and intensify their color. The neck, face, hands, and in fact all the body zones that are the most exposed, are the first to be affected. Our melanocytes start to react in an irregular way as do all the natural defenses of our skin. The least shock, the tiniest scratch, can leave indelible marks on the skin, which is why "spontaneous hematomas" become so common on old skin. Scars become more pronounced, as the elastic fibers of our skin become altered and the number of platelets (responsible for blood coagulation) grow fewer.

Once our skin has lost its tonicity, it quite literally spreads its surface, falling into folds and accentuating wrinkles. Finally, hormonal fluctuations are also related to this phenomenon, especially in the case of hyperpigmentation, and women are the most vulnerable.

What are the different types of wrinkles?

There are three types of wrinkles:

- *Actinic wrinkles* are spread all over the face. They result from prolonged exposure to the sun.

- *Character wrinkles* are known as frown marks (between the eyebrows), crow's feet (at the corners of the eyes), interrogation wrinkles (on the forehead), and nasal furrows (around the mouth).

- *Sagging wrinkles and folds* are visible under the eyelids, around the jowls, the neck, and the fold of bitterness (the extensions beneath the corners of the lips).

How can we fight daily against aging skin?

Creams, milks, and lotions contain antioxidant nutrients and extracts of plants or fruits that allow us to delay the aging of the skin. True, they cannot make time stand still, but they do protect the skin from the sun's rays, keep a good level of hydration, stimulate new cells, and fight against the attacks of free radicals. Applied appropriately, the nutrients and plant extracts directly nourish the skin, thereby completing the action of the supplements taken orally.

Why is it necessary to reinforce the antioxidant defense system?

The skin is especially vulnerable to attack from free radicals. When the antioxidant defenses are depressed, a large number of the body's cells find themselves without protection against oxidant aggression. At the skin level, the attacks by free radicals unfortunately leave visible traces. Most notably, they attack collagen, the protein that gives our epidermis its suppleness. As a result, our skin ages prematurely and the wrinkles deepen. It is, therefore, essential to keep the skin permanently nourished with enough antioxidants. Creams rich in antioxidants (vitamins C and E, selenium, ginkgo) bring nutrition directly to the skin, allowing it to reinforce its natural defenses and help it effectively fight against free radicals.

What are the benefits of vitamin C?

Vitamin C is the most abundant antioxidant in the skin and is particularly important for repairing lesions caused by free radicals, preventing them from becoming cancerous or accelerating the aging process. But vitamin C does more than neutralize free radicals. It is also necessary for the synthesis of collagen, which diminishes considerably as we get older. The slowing down of microcirculation, which goes hand in hand with the passing years, deprives the cells of the vitamin C necessary for a normal synthesis of collagen. The appropriate application of vitamin C can substantially increase its availability for the production of collagen. Studies have shown that vitamin C multiplies the synthesis of collagen fivefold.

What are the other efficient antioxidants?

Vitamin E protects the skin from damage by ultraviolet light and the oxidation of fats, reduces wrinkles, and slows down the progression of the aging process. This mechanism can also apply to other botanical antioxidants. Pycnogenol, blueberries, ginkgo, and licorice have been successfully used in this way as antioxidants. Studies have shown that they accelerate the healing of wounds and skin damaged by circulation problems.

What is "aesthetics without surgery"?

Aesthetic medicine now allows us to repair the ravages of time. Techniques without surgery can restore the bloom to your face: laser treatments, exfoliations, and injections are used alone or in combination to produce a face without wrinkles or scars. These methods can be used to correct acne scars, skin irregularities, and dilated pores.

However, actinic wrinkles are treated by different methods. I remove character lines and sagging folds by using resurfacing techniques, filling in wrinkles with hyaluronic acid (a lubricating substance that occurs naturally in the body) and Botox injections.

What does an injection consist of?

Injections are intended to fill in wrinkles that have been caused by the loss of tonicity in the skin and muscles. The products that are injected into these places can be put into two broad categories: those that are slowly resorbed and those that are quickly resorbed. These techniques are used in the treatment of deep wrinkles.

How does an injection of rapidly resorbed product work?

The procedure takes place at the doctor's office, where he or she injects collagen (either heterologous, coming from a different organism, or autologous, when it is your own collagen collected from elsewhere in your body) or hyaluronic acid into the furrow of a wrinkle. The advantage of injections is the absence of secondary effects (slight redness), but the effect wears off after six months or a year. Another technique consists of injecting fat into the wrinkles—this is called lipofilling or lipostructure, in which deep injections restore volume to your face.

How does an injection of slowly resorbed product work?

The doctor can also choose to apply a product that cannot be resorbed. With this method, the results will last for several years. The techniques for filling in wrinkles sometimes cause a small red patch or a bruise at the point of injection. It is always recommended during the hours following the procedure to abstain from laughing or eating, in order to allow the product to settle correctly into the wrinkle. A few days after the procedure, once the product is in place, the wrinkles that have been filled in will disappear.

If you want to sustain the effect, you must repeat the injections, because eventually the injected substances leave the site of the injection and are absorbed into the blood. Not all the products behave in the same way. Personally, I don't use these products; I only inject hyaluronic acid. This is my choice and it suits both me and my patients.

How can we make the results of injections last?

There's not much to do. It is recommended that you take care of the skin using cosmetics to prevent the appearance of new wrinkles. It is better to avoid exposure to the sun and any significant change in weight.

What is Botox?

Since its recent launch on the market, Botox has become a big star. It is a toxin used notably in the treatment of squints and migraines.

Botox makes wrinkles disappear by temporarily paralyzing the muscles that create them.

Through repeated use, certain facial movements, such as frowning, blinking, and wrinkling the nose reinforce the muscles responsible: this is how character lines develop. Crow's feet, the wrinkles on the forehead, and the lines between the eyebrows fall into this category. The corrective treatment specially designed for the character lines of the eyes and the forehead attack the source of the problem: the muscles.

Botox is a tool for weakening the muscles causing wrinkles in the upper part of the face. This substance is produced by the bacteria *Clostridium botulinum,* and then purified and extracted. The doctor injects small quantities of the toxin into the muscle. By rejuvenating the face, Botox gives it a more relaxed, serene, and rested appearance. It is a safe and efficient way of correcting wrinkles. Two annual injections are usually recommended to keep the relevant muscles inactive.

The procedure itself takes about fifteen minutes. It is not painful, although you feel a faint burning sensation for a few minutes at the place where the injection was made. In the hours that follow, you should avoid moving your facial muscles and take care not to use moisturizing creams, so that the product is not diffused into neighboring muscles.

What are the results?

The beneficial effects, though noticeable within seventy-two hours after treatment, reach their peak about ten days later. After four days, you can no longer move your eyebrows, but it is not until two weeks have passed that the muscles are really stabilized and the skin taut. You still keep your facial expressions since the doses are calculated so that the injected zone is never frozen and motionless.

Botox works for four to six months. You then need to repeat the injections twice a year to maintain the results. The sessions will gradually become further apart, because the Botox lasts longer each time. Gradually, you lose the habit of frowning and creasing your forehead. This method is useful in two ways: it cures wrinkles and also prevents the formation of character lines.

Isn't Botox dangerous?

The *Clostridium* bacteria produces a toxin that, absorbed in quantity, can cause botulism, a form of food poisoning. It would require a dose at least a thousand times higher than that used for treating wrinkles. By comparison, aspirin, although recognized as a safe form of medicine, can be fatal if the dose taken is ten times higher than recommended. Botox, therefore, has a much bigger security margin than most drugs.

Is Botox the best solution for wrinkles?

Specially conceived to reduce character lines, Botox acts on the muscles beneath the skin, but it will not necessarily modify all the wrinkles on the surface. There are other methods of reducing these wrinkles, such as collagen injections, Gore-Tex plastic implants, exfoliation, fat injections, and laser treatments. Ask your doctor to guide you to the solution that is most appropriate for your particular skin problem.

How can I get rid of blotches, brown marks, and little wrinkles?

All the small imperfections of the skin—blotches, age spots, or birth marks—can be erased for a long time by using laser treatment. This requires no anaesthetic and no drugs. Two treatment sessions of between five and twenty minutes is all it takes. There are two principal laser techniques to reduce, or even get rid of, wrinkles and other scars. These procedures require neither anesthetic nor hospitalization.

With resurfacing, the laser works on the upper parts of the wrinkle layer by layer (several microns deep), and the resulting smoothness makes it disappear after only a few sessions. In some case, the treatment can provoke postoperative irritation (red patches, erythema) for a few days, but it has no secondary effects and leaves no marks or discoloration. Two forms of laser are prescribed: one for deep wrinkles and scars, and the other for smaller facial wrinkles. The results are excellent in both cases and visible after one or two months.

Dermosurfacing is a new technique for combating wrinkles. It doesn't wear away the skin (so doesn't cause redness) but stimulates, through the thermic under-skin action of the laser, the production of collagen (constituting part of the skin). The treatment is completely

TIPS FOR SUCCESS

- Drink lots of water to ensure better hydration.

- Don't smoke, and consume alcohol in moderation.

- Complement your diet with nutrients that are beneficial to the skin.

- Clean your face gently, avoiding harsh soaps and water that is too hard.

- Avoid rubbing your skin when you apply cosmetics. Touch it gently instead.

- Make sure that all injected products used are from a reputable source, and remember that they must, for legal reasons, be used only in a medical environment.

natural and the results are visible after a few days—the skin is tauter and the wrinkles gone.

What is exfoliation?

Exfoliation, or peeling, is a chemical procedure that aims to wear away from the skin's surface the imperfections linked to aging. We distinguish, according to the depth of the skin treated, between light, medium, and deep exfoliation: all must be performed by an experienced doctor or in a special clinic for deep and extensive exfoliation. The results last between six months and a year, depending on the depth of the exfoliation. However, some wrinkles will always remain impervious to exfoliation, such as the vertical line between the eyebrows or the nasal furrows (leading from the nose to the corners of the lips), because they are due, in part, to the natural contraction of the muscles.

CHAPTER 12

The Essential Check-Up

JULIEN: *What is an evaluation of biological age?*

DR. CHAUCHARD: An evaluation of physiological, or biological, age is the first step you need to take in dealing with aging. Wanting to intervene in a process as complex as aging requires a global approach to our physiological systems. Measuring physiological age allows us to have an objective idea of how an individual is actually aging through evaluating a certain number of systems: vascular, cardiac, cerebral, neurosensory, bone, fatty mass, lean mass, and others.

Our physiological systems start to deteriorate from around age eighteen to twenty, without us really noticing. For example, our arteries, in the twenty years from age twenty to forty, increase their rigidity by around 50 percent. And increased rigidity does not mean they are "diseased." Arterial disease can happen much later. We can measure this arterial rigidity and so have a very precise idea of our stage of arterial aging. Accelerated aging means that at fifty years old we may have the arteries of someone of sixty or seventy years. We can also lose 30 percent of our muscular mass between age fifty and seventy. The earlier we intervene, the greater chance we have of doing so effectively.

When should we have our first complete check-up?

We can take steps to control the aging process from any age, but our capacity for intervention will be much more limited if we intervene later in life—so the sooner, the better. The first phase of life, from birth to age eighteen or twenty, is the growth phase, an extraordinarily complex time during which a great number of mechanisms are put in place. At this age, we should develop good eating habits, and that is already something.

Then, from age twenty to thirty, we are in top form. It would be interesting to have a first test during this period, not for treatment, but just to know where we stand. Knowing the optimum physiological condition of an individual will allow us to have points of reference for the rest of life. We are seeing more and more young people of twenty-five years, who have been sent in by their parents of fifty, just to have this basic check-up for reference.

Today, we are still working according to averages. But from the second physiological age check-up, we can move away from averages because we have a point of reference. Being able to offer young people a physiological evaluation today seems a good idea to me.

The further we extend the parameters of this assessment, the greater chance we have of a successful intervention. Also, we need to evaluate people and test them biologically, to know if they are lacking in some vitamin, trace element, or hormone, and to then see how all that interacts in the body. Because here, too, we are all very unequal in physiological terms. What may work wonderfully for one person is doomed to failure with another, which is why it is so important to evaluate the parameters regularly.

What does a check-up consist of?

A check-up gives us a great deal of useful information to evaluate:

- The state of different health profiles of the body; in total, thirty-two profiles must function harmoniously.

- The risks of cellular aging and the degradation of the cell membranes linked to inflammation.

- The condition of the arteries and, therefore, the risks of arteriosclerosis and atherosclerosis, and related diseases.

- Problems due to poor diet or lack of physical exercise.

- Finally, the level of different hormone secretions, in order to prepare therapeutic substitutions.

To this check-up, we can add a biophysical evaluation, which is carried out using computerized equipment and takes into account blood pressure, respiratory capacity, flexibility, endurance, resistance, and strength. These tests are not yet widely available, but certain clinics are already offering them.

I would remind you again that anti-aging depends, first of all, on your own willingness. Each of us is free to choose not to undertake it, but bear in mind what you are then exposing yourself to a programmed aging process that may be more or less accelerated.

Finally, remember that no prescription can be given once and for all, applicable for all patients. Instead, we need to put in place a personalized program, put together by your doctor, who will establish it according to your needs.

What should be my priority?

With a simple blood test that checks levels of C-reactive protein (CRP) and fibrinogen, you can see whether or not you are exposed to chronic inflammatory reactions and, therefore, accelerated aging. Add to that a check on oxidative stress in your body and you will know your "redox" situation, that is, the balance between the oxidant aggressors and the antioxidant defenses. These two tests are generally quite affordable.

The Golden Age

It's not that I'm scared of dying,
I just don't want to be there when it happens.

—WOODY ALLEN

The medical world doesn't talk much about the possibilities of controlling aging. Hardly surprising, in these conditions, that few people seek to cure this general decline. We say that aging is normal, and for some people it even has a certain beauty. The evolution of our vital equilibrium requires a particular and complete treatment, a total reorganization of our health routine and the control of our "health capital."

The right person to advise you must be an expert in several subjects. A book is first of all the scene of a meeting: the author writes for his reader. I speak to those who believe, like Epictetus, that "living is not a good thing but what is a good thing is living well."

How old are we? We are constantly talking about the problems of growing old when there are plenty of elderly people in top physical form. At the other extreme, there are men not yet forty years of age who are suffering from premature impotence, excess weight, and therefore a loss of equilibrium.

What age is the mature adult, the one we are talking about in this book? You may want to be given an average figure age range, but is there an average age? I would like this expression to be read like a generic title. Balzac's famous novel *A Woman of Thirty* described the condition of a woman who had been married for a certain time and who was suffering from a crisis of lost illusions. According to Balzac, a woman of thirty wasn't exactly thirty years old, or thirty-five, or even fifty! In the same way, "the aging person" who wants to control aging concerns individuals of thirty years as well as septuagenarians. Every man and every woman has their own body, and each has its own aging pattern. No two are the same!

THE STRENGTH OF NATURE VARIES

Are all persons born equal? Legally, yes. But when it comes to potential vitality, let's not begin the old debate of nature versus nurture. Education, environment, socio-professional milieu, and historical period are all undeniably factors in our inequality in life. In the Middle Ages, a man rarely lived beyond the age of forty. In the twenty-first century, people hope to get to know their great-great-grandchildren. Such is the privilege of a person who lives in a healthy environment where hygiene is normal and infections rare. And even luckier for the person if he or she has a job that doesn't involve physical hardship.

But living with a healthy mind and spirit does not confer immortality. Nature also has certain rights, and aging sooner or later will affect people according to their own heredity or constitution. Different stages of controlling aging correspond to these different sorts of individuals. In concrete terms, a yearly check-up will indicate a lowering or other disruption in the hormone levels, and so equilibrium can be reestablished, thereby preventing any repercussions to the body as a whole.

THE REAL LIFE INSURANCE

Whether you are suffering from aging, or simply taking precautions, it is in everyone's interest to master the aging process through hormone control. However, few people take such measures to improve their health and vitality. Why? Because few people take care of their aging process.

For more than twenty years now, I have been subscribing annually to a life insurance policy. The older I get, the more money accrues, which will fall to my heirs one day when I die. An altruistic gesture, a sign of love—life insurance deserves these encomiums. And yet it needs to be pointed out that it is not my life that is insured, but the comfort and happiness of other lives. I subscribe in the full understanding that this is the "life insurance of my heirs." And it is with equal lack of hesitation that I insure elsewhere my own life with my "health capital."

Controlling the aging of the body, because it constitutes a complete health program, can be seen as the real life insurance. Insuring our life can become as simple as insuring our home. Thinking of our health when we should, and the way we should, also means we don't need to think about it nervously after each overindulgent meal.

Tomorrow's person is well-informed, takes precautions, and controls his or her aging. Tomorrow's doctor will no longer be merely required to cure, his or her role will become preventive.

LIVING IN THE GOLDEN AGE

The Roman poet Propertius recounts the mythical succession of generations of men, from the "golden race" to the "iron race." All those who have studied a little Latin at school will no doubt remember the version of the poem on the golden age, and the difficulty of translating the literary expression "the youth of old men." In the golden age, men remained young until the end of their lives. The poem cites healthy lifestyle as the cause and reason for this "lifelong youth": men eat fruit, make love all day in secret caves, and cultivate flowers and the trust of the gods.

The myth, like all myths, takes its origin and motivation from popular desire—the desire to live in good health throughout our lives. To counteract the fatality of human nature, prodigal in sickness and death, the ancient poets used to write about the golden age. Today, information has taken over from poetry, and medicine has taken over from desire.

It is not a foolish dream to talk about a healthy old age. The control of glycation or oxidation is less astonishing than nuclear power, trips to the moon, or genetic modification. We are talking here about maintaining our bodies and learning to control our aging, just as we teach our children the basics of hygiene: washing, brushing our teeth, watching what we eat, and so on.

Each society teaches health and hygiene, and the things we learn develop and refine these healthy conditions almost to perfection. Let us take one example of socio-medical information that is quite revolutionary: when Mao Tse-tung came to power in China at the end of the 1940s, he made the death rate fall simply by informing people about the importance of cutting their fingernails, which shows how catastrophic hygiene conditions had caused a shockingly high death rate. When you consider how much cardiovascular disease costs our healthcare system, the treatments that I outline ought to be undertaken by the state.

Our grandparents died, on average, twenty years younger than our parents. We may live twenty years longer than them. But in what condition—in a wheelchair, bedridden? No one wants to simply "last" twenty years longer. The question of the golden age is the desire to live for a long time but in top physical and mental form. Utopia? No, it is not science fiction, but it hasn't yet taken place for us, common mortals that we are. Tens of thousands of people are living today who are more than 100 years old; there will be hundreds of thousands in the next century.

The golden age cannot be achieved by simply taking a pill. We are not talking about an artificial paradise. No form of treatment makes sense unless it goes hand in hand with a healthy life, including a balanced diet and exercise.

FEELING GOOD IN YOURSELF

The golden age is frequently misinterpreted: living for a long time and in good health does not mean taking on the appearance of a young person of twenty-five years and staying that way until the day you die. The main objective of age-prevention treatment is the health of each and every one of us. Certainly, a person in top form may be more "aesthetically pleasing" than a doddery old person, but the perverse use of treatment is a temptation that must be avoided. The goal of the balanced use of my method is good health; its deviation would be a treatment with which to "dope" patients.

Let us remember the story of *The Picture of Dorian Gray.* Oscar Wilde's famous story concerns a young dandy who sells his soul to the devil in exchange for a considerable favor: to remain young right up until his death. Behind the angelic face that Dorian Gray displays right up until his dying day, another face is hiding—that of an old man debauched by what he has really become. This other face cannot be hidden. This is the moral of the story, which is revealed to us at the end in a portrait of Dorian Gray that has aged catastrophically. All the would-be Dorian Grays who think that a few pills will give them the energy of a man of twenty-five are heading for disaster.

I have treated a great many men and women and the experience has led me to this conclusion: in order to live better for longer, we must incorporate this desire into our lifestyle. That way, our will to succeed blends with the dream and nothing seems too difficult.

So now it's up to you to think about it and take action. Life is not a dress rehearsal during which we may correct our mistakes. Do it today, this book will help you. Go on, take heart, and start right away on this program to look and feel younger. I would be so pleased to share your joy!

Resources

A number of associations offer information, advice, and services for those dealing with particular health problems.

ALCOHOLISM

Alcoholics Anonymous (AA)

Grand Central Station
P.O. Box 459
New York, NY 10163
Website: www.alcoholics-
anonymous.org

State and local AA groups can be found on the AA Website or your Yellow Pages directory.

CANCER

American Cancer Society

Telephone: 1-800-227-2345
Website: www.cancer.org

HEART DISEASE

American Heart Association

National Center
7272 Greenville Avenue
Dallas, TX 75231
Telephone: 1-800-242-8721
Website: www.amhrt.org

DIABETES

American Diabetes Association

Attn: National Call Center
1701 North Beauregard Street
Alexandria, VA 22311
Telephone: 1-800-342-2383
Website: www.diabetes.org

References

Adams, P. B., S. Lawson, et al. "Arachidonic Acid to Eicosapentaenoic Acid Ratio in Blood Correlates Positively with Clinical Symptoms of Depression." *Lipids* 31:Suppl (1996): S157–S161.

Al, M., A. C. van Houwelingen, et al. "Long-chain Polyunsaturated Fatty Acids, Pregnancy, and Pregnancy Outcome." *Am J Clin Nutr* 71:1 Suppl (2000): 285S–291S.

Alarcon de la Lastra, C., M. D. Barranco, V. Motilva, and J. M. Herrerias. "Mediterranean Diet and Health: Biological Importance of Olive Oil." *Curr Pharm Des* 7:10 (2001): 933–950.

Anonymous. "*Centella asiatica* (Gotu kola). Botanical Monograph." *Am J Nat Med* 3:6 (1996): 22.

Baulieu, E., G. Thomas, et al. "Dehydroepiandrosterone (DHEA), DHEA Sulfate, and Aging: Contribution of the DHEAga Study to a Socio-biochemical Issue." *Proc Natl Acad Sci USA* 97:8 (2000): 4279–4284.

Beaser, S. B., and T. B. Massel. "Therapeutic Evaluation of Testosterone in Peripheral Vascular Disease." *New Engl J Med* (1942).

Benton, D. "The Impact of the Supply of Glucose to the Brain on Mood and Memory." *Nutr Rev* 59:1 Part 2 (2001): S20–S21.

Berdanier, C. D. *Advanced Nutrition: Micronutrients.* Boca Raton, FL: CRC Press, 1998.

Bianchini, P., B. Osima, M. S. Cetino, et al. Sostanze Biologicomente Attive in Astratti di Placenta, Nestre Central Library at Vevey, March 1977.

Bierhaus, A., et al. "Advanced Glycation and Product-induced Activation of NF-kappa B Is Suppressed by Alpha-lipoic Acid in Cultured Andothetial Cells." *Diabetes* 46:9 (1997): 1481–1490.

Charry, Michel. "The Revolutionary Process of Rejuvenation." *Ambiance de Paris* 47–48 (October 1979).

Chen, L., J. Tang, et al. "The Effect of Location of Transcutaneous Electrical Nerve Stimulation of Postoperative Opioid Analgesic Requirement: Acupoint versus Nonacupoint Stimulation." *Anesth Analg* 87 (1998): 1129–1134.

Choi, S., W. Son, et al. "The Wound-healing Effect of a Glycoprotein Fraction Isolated from Aloe Vera." *Br J Dermatol* 145:4 (2001): 535–545.

Christman, J. W., T. S. Blackwell, and B. H. Juurlink. "Redox Regulation of Nuclear Factor Kappa B: Therapeutic Potential for Attenuating Inflammatory Responses." *Brain Pathol* 10:1 (2000): 153–162.

Cole, A. C., E. M. Gisoldi, and R. M. Grossman. "Clinical and Consumer Evaluations of Improved Facial Appearance After 1 Month Use of Topical Dimethylaminoethanol." Poster presentation, American Academy of Dermatology, February 22–26, 2002, New Orleans, Louisiana.

———. "Long-term Safety and Efficacy Evaluation of a New Skip Firming Technology, Dimethylaminoethanol." Poster presentation, American Academy of Dermatology, February 22–26, 2002, New Orleans, Louisiana.

D'Angelo, S., C. Manna, V. Migliardi, et al. "Pharmacokinetics and Metabolism of Hydroxytyrosol, A Natural Antioxidant from Olive Oil." *Drug Metab Dispos* 29:11 (2001): 1492–1498.

Day, R. V. "Male Sex Hormone Therapy." *J Urol* (1939).

De Lorgeril, M., S. Renaud, et al. "Mediterranean Alpha-linoleic Acid Rich Diet in Secondary Prevention of Coronary Heart Disease." *The Lancet* 343 (1994): 1454–1459.

DiLorenzo, T. M., E. P. Bargman, et al. "Long-term Effects of Aerobic Exercise on Psychological Outcomes." *Prevent Med* 28:1 (1999): 75–85.

Duan, W., and M. P. Mattson. "Dietary Restriction and 2-deoxyglucose Administration Improve Behavioral Outcome and Reduce Degeneration of Dopaminergic Neurons in Models of Parkinson's Disease." *J Neurosci Res* 57:2 (1999): 195–206.

Eidelsberg, J. "The Male Sex Hormone." *Med Clin North Am* (1938).

Fairfield, K. M., and R. H. Fletcher. "Vitamins for Chronic Disease Prevention in Adults: Scientific Review." *JAMA* 287:23 (2002): 3116–3126.

Filatov, V. *The Therapeutic Tissues.* Moscow: Foreign Language Editions, 1955.

Food and Nutrition Board, Institute of Medicine. *Dietary Reference Intakes: A Risk Assessment Model for Establishing Upper Intake Levels for Nutrients.* Washington, D.C.: National Academy Press, 1999.

Gismondo, M. R., L. Drago, M. Fassina, et al. "Immunostimulating Effect of Oral Glutamine." *Digest Dis Sci* 43:8 (1998): 1752–1754.

Hagen, T. M., J. Liu, J. Lykkesfeldt, et al. "Feeding Acetyl-L-carnitine and Lipoic Acid to Old Rats Significantly Improves Metabolic Function While Decreasing Oxidative Stress." *Proc Natl Acad Sci USA* 99:4 (2002): 1870–1875.

Haker, E., H. Egekvist, et al. "Effect of Sensory Stimulation (Acupuncture) on Sympathetic and Parasympathetic Activities in Healthy Subjects." *J Anatomic Nerv Syst* 79:1 (2000): 52–59.

He, D., J. Berg, et al. "Effects of Acupuncture on Smoking Cessation or Reduction for Motivated Smokers." *Prevent Med* 26 (1997): 208–214.

Hibbeln, J. R. "Long-chain Polyunsaturated Fatty Acids in Depression and Related Conditions." In M. Peet, I. Glen, and D. Horrobin, *Phospholipid Spectrum Disorder* (Lancashire, England: Marius Press, 1999), 195–210.

Holt, S. H., J. C. Miller, and P. Peroez. "An Insulin Index of Foods: The Insulin Demand Generated by 1000-kj Portions of Common Foods." *Am J Clin Nutr* 66:5 (1997): 1264–1276.

Iselin, M. P., and Martin Gossel. "Our Experience of Tissue Therapy." *Memoir of the Academy of Surgery* 16117 (1953).

Iselin, Martin, and Michel Charry. "Is It Possible to Defeat Old Age?" *Ambiance de Paris* 51–52 (December 1971).

Jentzer, A., and J. J. Kobel. "Amino Acids in the Post- and Pre-operatory Periods." *Experimental Medicine and Surgery* 12 (1953).

Kagan, V. E., A. Shvedova, E. Serbinova, et al. "Dihydrolipoic Acid—A Universal Antioxidant Both in the Membrane and in the Aqueous Phase. Reduction of Preoxyl, Ascorbyl and Chromanoxyl Radicals." *Biochem Pharmacol* 44:8 (1992): 1637–1649.

LaRoche, G., H. Simmonet, and E. Bompard. "Appreciation by Quantitative Tests of the Effects of the Male Hormone on Elderly Men." *Bull Acad Med Paris* (1938).

Lausseure, M. "Tissue Therapy in Stomatology." *Annals of Histotherapy* 10 (April 1952).

Leibenluft, E., P. L. Fiero, and D. R. Rubinow. "Effects of the Menstrual Cycle on Dependent Variables in Mood Disorder Research." *Arch Gen Psychiatr* 51:10 (1994): 761–781.

Li, Y., G. Tougas, et al. "The Effects of Acupuncture on Gastrointestinal Function and Disorders." *Am J Gastroenterol* 87 (1992): 1372–1381.

Lin, Y., M. W. Rajala, J. P. Berger, et al. "Hyperglycemia-induced Production of Acute Phase Reactants in Adipose Tissue." *J Biol Chem* 276:45 (2001): 42077–42083.

Liu, K., J. Stamler, et al. "Dietary Lipids, Sugar, Fiber, and Mortality from Coronary Heart Disease—Bivariate Analysis of International Data." *Artherosclerosis* 2 (1982): 221–227.

Maes, M., R. Smith, et al. "Fatty Acid Composition in Major Depression: Decreased w3 Fractions in Cholesteryl Esters and Increased C20:4 Omega 6/C20:5 Omega-3 Ratio in Cholesteryl Esters and Phospholipids." *J Affect Disord* 38 (1996): 35–46.

Marshall, B. "The *Campylobacter pylori* Story." *Scand J Gastroenterol* 146:Suppl (1988): 58–66.

Martinez-Dominguez, E., R. de la Puerta, and V. Ruiz-Gutierrez. "Protective Effects upon Experimental Inflammation Models of a Polyphenol-supplemented Virgin Olive Oil Diet." *Inflamm Res* 50:2 (2001): 102–106.

Medalie, J. H., K. C. Stange, et al. "The Importance of Bio-psychosocial Factors in the Development of Duodenal Ulcer in a Cohort of Middle-aged Men." *Am J Epidemiol* 136:10 (1992): 1280–1287.

Meyer, M., H. L. Pahl, and P. A. Baeuerle. "Regulation of the Transcription Factors NF-kappa B and AP-1 by Redox Changes." *Chem Biol Interact* 91:2–3 (1994): 91–100.

Milad, M., and G. I. Quirk. "Neurons in Medial Prefrontal Cortex Signal Memory for Fear Extinction." *Nature* 420 (2002): 70–74.

Nemets, B., Z. Stahl, et al. "Addition of Omega-3 Fatty Acid to Maintenance Medication Treatment for Recurrent Unipolar Depressive Disorder." *Am J Psychiatr* 159 (2002): 477–479.

Newerla, G. J. "The History of the Discovery and Isolation of the Male Hormone." *New England Journal of Medicine* (1943).

Pawlak, D. B., J. M. Bryson, G. S. Denyer, and J. C. Brand-Miller. "High

Glycemic Index Starch Promotes Hyper-secretion of Insulin and Higher Body Fat in Rats Without Affecting Insulin Sensitivity." *J Nutr* 131:1 (2001): 99–104.

Pert, C. B., H. E. Dreher, et al. "The Psychosomatic Network: Foundations of Mind-Body Medicine." *Altern Ther Health Med* 4:4 (1998): 30–41.

Renaud, S., M. Ciavatti, et al. "Protective Effects of Dietary Calcium and Magnesium on Platelet Function and Atherosclerosis in Rabbits Fed Saturated Fat." *Atherosclerosis* 47 (1983): 189–198.

Reynolds, P., P. T. Boyd, et al. "The Relationship Between Social Ties and Survival Among Black and White Breast Cancer Patients. National Cancer Institute Black/White Cancer Survival Study Group." *Cancer Epidemiol Biomarkers Prev* 3:3 (1994): 253–259.

Roman, R. J. "P-450 Metabolites of Arachinodic Acid in the Control of Cardiovascular Function." *Physiol Rev* 82:1 (2002): 131–185.

Serbinova, E. A., and L. Packer. "Antioxidant Properties of Alpha-tocopherol and Alpha-tocotrienol." *Method Enzymol* 234 (1994): 354–366.

Serbinova, E., V. Kagan, D. Han, and L. Packer. "Free Radical Recycling and Intramembrane Mobility in the Antioxidant Properties of Alpha-tocopherol and Alpha-tocotrienol." *Free Radic Biol Med* 10:5 (1991): 263–275.

Soulie de Morant, G. L. *L'acupuncture Chinoise.* Paris: Maloine Éditeurs, 1972.

Stoll, A. L. *The Omega-3 Connection: The Groundbreaking Omega-3 Antidepression Diet and Brain Program.* New York: Simon & Schuster, 2001.

Storby, B., and M. Nichool. *The LCP Solution: The Remarkable Nutritional Treatment for ADHD, Dyslexia, and Dyspraxia.* New York: Ballantine Books, 2000.

Wertheimer, Gauthier and Marek. *On Treatment for Tissue, According to the Procedure of Filatov.* Paris: La Presse Médicale, April 1948.

Wilson, S., L. Becker, et al. "Fifteen-month Follow-up of Eye Movement Desensitization and Reprocessing (EMDR) Treatment for Posttraumatic Stress Disorder and Psychological Trauma." *J Consult Clin Psych* 65:6 (1997): 1047–1056.

Zs-Nagy, I. "The Membrane Hypothesis of Aging: Its Relevance to Recent Progress in Genetic Research." *J Mol Med* 75:10 (1997): 703–714.

Zs-Nagy, I., and I. Semsei. "Centrophenoxine Increases the Rates of Total and mRNA Synthesis in the Brain Cortex of Old Rats: An Explanation of Its Action in Terms of the Membrane Hypothesis of Aging." *Exp Gerontol* 19:3 (1984): 171–178.

Zs-Nagy, I., R. G. Cutler, and I. Semsei. "Dysdifferentiation Hypothesis of Aging and Cancer. A Comparison with the Membrane Hypothesis of Aging." *Ann NY Acad Sci* 521 (1988): 215–225.

Zurrow, H., G. Saland, C. Klein, and S. Goldman. "The Effect of Testosterone Proportionate in the Treatment of Arteriosclerosis." *J Lab Clin Med* (1942).

Index

P

Palm of the hand test, 40
Pancreas, 34, 42, 98, 99, 101, 107
Parkinson's disease, 67
Perls, Thomas, 41
Physical activity. _See_ Exercise.
Picture of Dorian Gray, The
    (Wilde), 133
PMS. _See_ Premenstrual
    syndrome.
Pores, 120
Potassium, 68
Poultry, 95, 113
Premenstrual syndrome, 87, 88
Pressure cookers, 110
Propertius, 131
Prostaglandins, 84
Proteins, 31, 34, 35, 47, 49,
    51–52, 95, 98, 99, 101, 103,
    109, 111, 115
Psoriasis, 82
Purslane, 87
Pycnogenol, 120

R

Resurfacing, 123
Retina, 76
Rice, 44, 45, 48, 113

S

Salad Nicoise, 36
Salt, 110
Scars, 118
    acne, 120
Sclerosis, 89
Seeds, 49
Selenium, 63, 64, 65, 67, 68, 69,
    71, 119

Shellfish, 103, 113
Silicium, 68
Skin, 40, 62, 74, 84, 117–124
Smoking, 27, 67, 84, 90–91, 96,
    124
Snacks, 34, 36, 47, 99, 101,
    103, 112, 115
SOD. _See_ Superoxide
    dismutase.
Soft drinks, 46, 51
Soy, 109, 113
Spices, 107
Spinach, 71
Spirulina, 82
Starch, 98, 99, 102
Stecker's degradation, 73
Stomach, 98, 99
Stress, 84, 90, 91, 100, 115–116
Strokes, 67
Sugar, 42, 43, 44, 45, 48, 98,
    101, 102, 109
Sulfur, 69
Sunlight, 118, 120, 121
Superoxide dismutase, 32, 64

T

Taurine, 63
Tea, 34, 51, 107, 108, 112, 113
30-Day Timely Nutrition Vitality
    Program, 95, 96, 97–116
    rules, 101–102
Thrombosis, 94
Time, 98–100
    afternoon, 99
    evening, 99–100
    midday, 99, 193
    morning, 98–99, 103
Tocopherols. _See_ Vitamin E.

About the Author

Dr. Claude Chauchard obtained his doctorate in medicine, biology, and sports medicine from the University of Montpellier, France. He is the founder of the International Institute for Preventive Anti-Ageing Medicine and was an Assistant Professor at the University of Montpellier from 1974 to 1979. He is also one of the world's top specialists in preventive medicine for aging, and the first to introduce this concept in Asia. Over one million copies of his twelve books on the aging process have been sold. He gives regular lectures and seminars in Paris, Milan, Barcelona, Brussels, Monte Carlo, Rio de Janeiro, Geneva, and other major cities around the world.